UNPROCESS

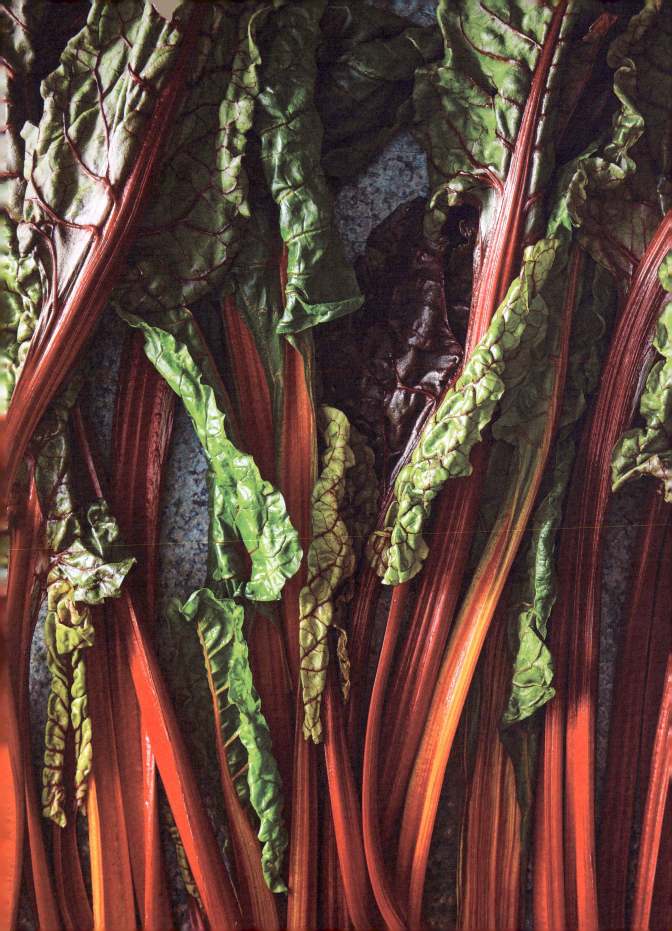

UNPROCESS

The 30-Day Challenge

Jason Adetola Mackson

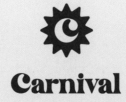

Carnival

CONTENTS

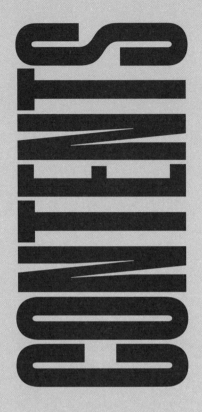

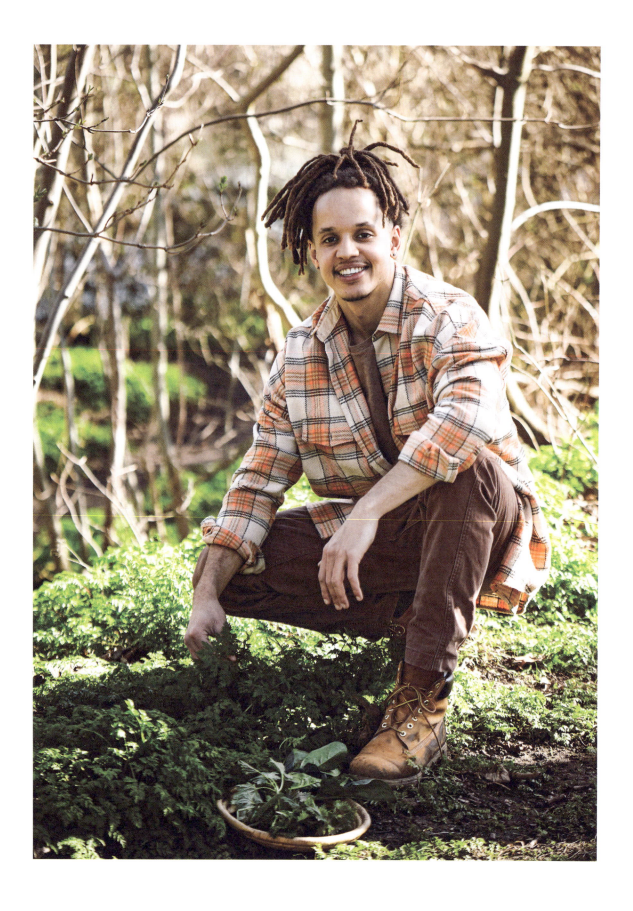

INTRODUCTION

Unprocess: The 30-Day Whole Food Challenge

... something is shifting. We are starting to regain an understanding of the spiritual, physical and emotional importance of food – from its contribution to longevity, to its influence on the quality of life.

We live in a time where convenience has taken priority over nourishment. Ultra-processed foods fill our shelves, meals are designed for shelf life instead of sustaining life, and the link between what we eat and how we feel has been lost. Nature designed us for a way of eating and living that has all but disappeared from modern culture. We now see food as a quick fix – something to curb hunger, to be counted in calories, to be squeezed into our schedules, rather than recognising it as an internal compass guiding us to our birthright: health and happiness.

But something is shifting. We are starting to regain an understanding of the spiritual, physical and emotional importance of food – from its contribution to longevity, to its influence on the quality of life. The body is an intelligent system, finely tuned for survival and reproduction. In our natural environment, what feels good is good. That's how nature ensures we eat what serves us and stops us when we've had enough.

But what happens when we take food out of its natural context? Think of an apple – how many whole apples could you pick and eat in one sitting before your body signalled that you'd had enough? Four? Maybe five? Now, what if those apples were juiced, stripped of their fibre and concentrated with added sugars? Suddenly, consuming the equivalent of 15, even 20 apples in liquid form feels effortless. When we alter food from its whole form, we bypass our body's natural regulatory system – the signals designed to maintain balance and prevent overconsumption.

Let's take another great example: potatoes. How many plain, boiled or steamed potatoes could you eat in one sitting? Two? Maybe three? There's a natural stopping point. Your body recognises the density, the fibre and the sheer volume of the food and signals you to slow down. What happens when those same potatoes are deep-fried, coated in processed seed oils and sprinkled with table salt? Suddenly, that natural stopping point is overridden. The crispy texture, the high fat content and the stimulating combination of salt and sweetness – often from ketchup or other condiments – make it easy to eat an entire plate of chips (fries) without even thinking.

This is what happens when food is stripped from its natural state, manipulated for hyper-palatability and engineered for excessive stimulation. It doesn't just change how it tastes – it changes how our body perceives it. We have numbed ourselves to the pleasure of whole natural foods; we no longer eat in response to hunger; we eat in response to the excessive stimulation of processed foods, which override the very mechanisms that evolved to protect us.

The modern diet has distanced us from the body's built-in monitoring system. What was once fresh, vibrant and whole is now refined, stripped and repackaged into something convenient but nutritionally hollow. And, as a result, we've normalised fatigue, brain fog, bloating, obesity and chronic inflammation as just part of life.

But what if we stripped it all back? What if, for 30 days, we chose to eat only whole natural food – the kind that fuels, heals and sustains us? This book is your guide to doing exactly that.

This is not about restriction. It's not about following trends or chasing perfection. It's about returning to the way food was always meant to be – simple, unprocessed and deeply nourishing. Over the next 30 days, you'll experience what it feels like to fuel your body with the right foods, to break free from the cycle of processed convenience, and to rediscover the power of eating consistent with our natural history.

This is an invitation – not just to a challenge, but to a shift in the way you see healthy living.

> This is an invitation – not just to a challenge, but to a shift in the way you see healthy living.

Why 30 Days?

Change feels overwhelming when it's indefinite, but when you commit to something for just 30 days, it becomes doable. As Henry Ford said, 'Nothing is particularly hard if you divide it into small jobs.' The 30-Day Whole Food Challenge does just that – breaking it down step by step, making real nourishment simple, achievable and life-changing. And the best part? The results speak for themselves. More energy, better digestion, clearer skin, deeper sleep – these are just a few of the benefits people may experience when they step away from processed foods and eat in alignment with how we were biologically designed to thrive.

This book is not about eating 'clean' every single day or obsessing over rules. It's about forming habits that help you thrive long-term. And by the time you reach the end of these 30 days, you'll have a whole new understanding and inspiration for how to support your body with what it truly needs to feel its best.

Think of this as an experiment. Not a diet, but a reset. For one month, you'll remove what's been holding you back – processed, refined and artificial foods – and fuel your body with what it was designed to thrive on: fruit, vegetables, nuts, seeds, legumes, ancient grains and high-quality animal proteins (if you choose to include them). And, by the end, you won't just feel different – you'll see food differently.

My Journey

This book is the culmination of everything I've learned along the way. I want this book to help people, but it should not take the place of medical or nutritional advice from a trained professional, especially for individuals with diagnosed conditions such as cancer. It's about simplifying your approach to food, fuelling your body with real nourishment and feeling good – deeply, consistently and sustainably.

I didn't always eat this way. Like many, I once saw food as little more than calories, cravings and a means to an end. That all changed in 2016 when my mother was diagnosed with Hodgkins Lymphoma, an uncommon cancer that develops in the lymphatic system. Suddenly, it felt like my mother was no longer the narrator of her own story. A healthy person wants a million things, a sick person only wants one – to be healthy again. The cancer had spread throughout her lymph nodes. As a teenager, I felt helpless. But my mother's resilience, dedication and refusal to let the cancer dictate the outcome of her life inspired a shift in me and my family – one that would later impact thousands through my community, The Electric Tribe.

In the wake of her treatment, I became obsessed with understanding how food could aid healing and vitality. I started researching, questioning and experimenting. What I discovered was both simple and transformative – our bodies thrive when we nourish them the way nature intended. When we return to a diet rooted in real, whole foods, we sidestep the common pitfalls of modern eating – such as fatigue, obesity and digestive discomfort – that so many people accept as normal. Mum felt a big impact from making these dietary changes alongside her treatment – she felt she had more energy and focus, her fatigue improved.

Our kitchen transformed. Where it was once filled with quick fixes and processed convenience foods, it become a space of intention. Fresh produce replaced packaged goods. Fruits (the original candy) took the place of artificial sweets. Highly processed energy drinks were swapped for herbal infusions. Every meal was made with ingredients we could name, touch and trust. If we couldn't find it in nature, we didn't eat it.

What I discovered was both simple and transformative – our bodies thrive when we nourish them the way nature intended.

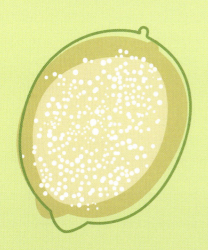

As I continued down this path, I saw just how disconnected most people had become from real nourishment. We live in a world where food is designed for profit and speed rather than sustenance. I started sharing what I was learning – posting recipes, and experiences online. What happened next changed everything.

The Birth of The Electric Tribe

At first, it was just me and my family experimenting with different foods to find what would help my mother regain her strength after cancer therapy. Every meal became a test, a lesson in how food could nourish the body. We swapped out what didn't serve her for what did, cutting out the processed, artificial and inflammatory foods and replacing them with the real, whole ingredients.

The changes my mother experienced were undeniable. As the weeks went by, she felt her energy returning and her mind became sharper. Watching this transformation unfold before my eyes at just 18 years old was the first time I truly understood the power of eating in alignment with our natural history. This wasn't just about her recovery anymore – it was about something much bigger.

What we had discovered wasn't complicated. It was intuitive, accessible and deeply rooted in the way humans can eat in harmony with nature. And yet, so many people had lost their way when it came to food. The more I learned, the more I felt an urgency to share. So, I started posting – simple swaps, whole-food alternatives, meals that left me feeling stronger, clearer and more energised. The recipes resonated with people. They reached out to say they weren't just eating better – they were feeling better. Their energy levels soared, digestion improved and some people who had struggled with their health for years suddenly felt like they had found a missing piece. It was clear: this wasn't just about food, it was about reclaiming our well-being and reconnecting with what it means truly to nourish ourselves.

What started as a few posts turned into a community. I called it The Electric Tribe – a space for people who wanted to unprocess their life, reconnect with nature and live with energy and vitality. From hosting supper clubs and foraging walks, to becoming a leader in the seaweed supplement industry, the response was undeniable. People were weren't looking for another diet or trend. They were looking for something real.

But The Electric Tribe has always been more than just a community – it's a movement. A return to balance, to nourishment, to living in sync with nature. It's a reminder that food is more than just fuel: it has the power to support recovery and wellbeing. No gimmicks. No complicated formulas. Just real food that works with your body, not against it.

It was clear: this wasn't just about food, it was about reclaiming our well-being and reconnecting with what it means truly to nourish ourselves.

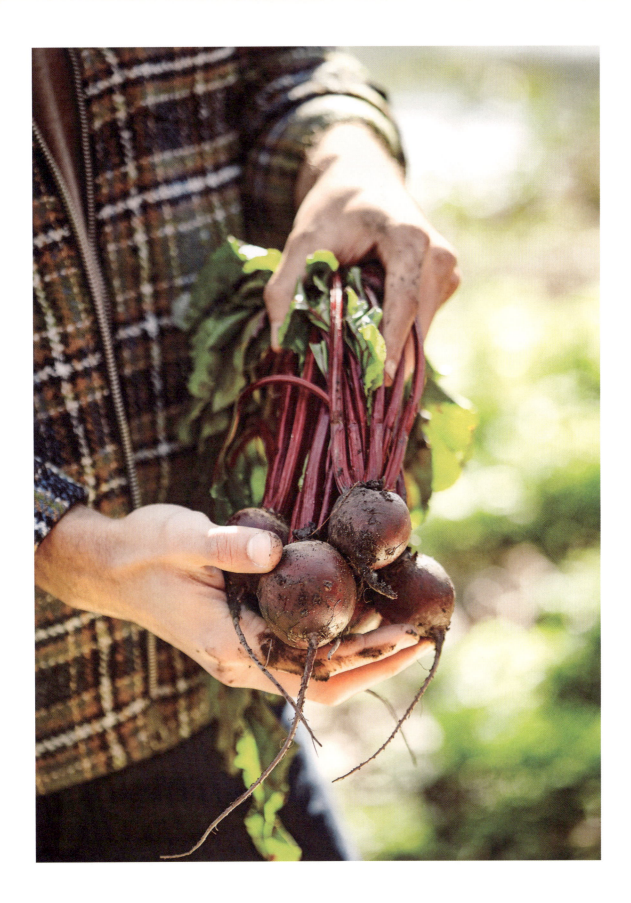

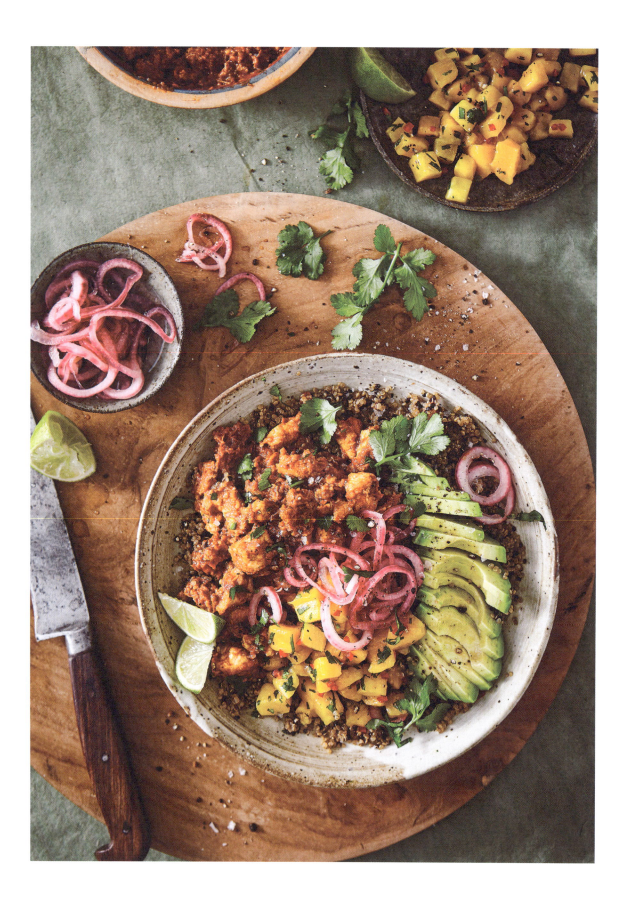

What You Will Find in the Book and How to Use It

Every recipe in this book has been crafted with care – designed to nourish, sustain and reconnect you with real ingredients.

- **Simple, whole-food recipes** that are easy-to-prepare, nutrient-dense, flavourful and designed to give you slowly-released, sustained energy.

- **Essential ingredients** – a carefully selected list of nutrient-rich whole foods, rooted in nature and that aim to support vitality and wellbeing.

- **A structured, step-by-step meal plan** to guide you through the 30-day challenge.

- **Nutritional insights** to help you understand how real food fuels your body.

- **Deeper connection** to food that nurtures not just your body, but also your mind and spirit – deepening your connection to yourself, nature and the world around you.

- **Sustainable habits** that go beyond the challenge, empowering you to maintain a whole-food lifestyle effortlessly.

Every recipe in this book has been crafted with care – designed to nourish, sustain and reconnect you with real ingredients. Real food is a conversation between your body and nature – these meals ensure that dialogue flows seamlessly and they work in sync with your body's blueprint for health. You won't find highly processed ingredients here. Just simple and effective nutrition that tastes incredible and leaves you feeling even better.

You can use this book as a simple cookbook. There are over 90 inspiring, delicious recipes to flick through and choose from whenever you feel the need. You can also use the recipes as part of a 30-day plan with suggested meal planners, lifestyle tips and guidance (see pages 188–199). Either way, there's something for everyone.

Left: Smoky Chipotle-Spiced Tofu (see page 88)

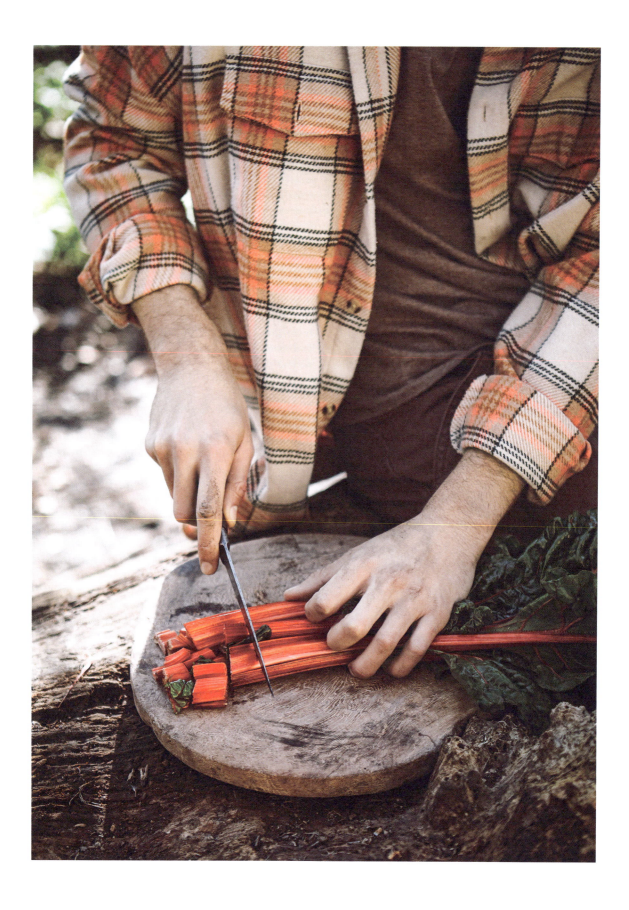

WHOLE FOODS FOUNDATION

What Are Whole Foods?

If humans disappeared tomorrow, what foods would remain in 10, 15, or even 100 years? Would energy drinks still flow from rivers? Would candy bars grow on trees? Would fields of white bread and cornflakes sprout from the earth? The answer is obvious. Whole foods are the ones that have always existed – the ones nature continues to provide, season after season, with or without us.

Whole foods are the foundation of nourishment – ingredients in their purest form, untouched by excessive refinement, artificial additives, or chemical alterations. They are fresh fruits and vegetables, whole grains, nuts, seeds, legumes and high-quality animal products in their most natural state. Unlike processed foods engineered for convenience, stimulation, and shelf life, whole foods are rich in the vitamins, minerals and phytonutrients our bodies instinctively thrive on. They are not just sustenance, they are nature's blueprint to operate at optimal capacity.

Why Whole Foods?

Have you ever seen an overweight animal in the wild? Animals in the wild don't waste energy – they move with purpose, efficiency and instinctive balance. Reptiles, for instance, bask in the sun to absorb heat instead of wasting energy generating their own body warmth. Unlike humans, wild animals maintain their health and fitness effortlessly, without counting calories or restricting portions. Even when food is abundant in their natural habitat, they eat intuitively, consuming just what they need for survival, energy and longevity. This instinctive regulation, known as satiation, ensures that animals in their natural environment remain lean, strong and vital.

For most of human history, we lived by this same principle. Our ancestors didn't track macros or debate diet trends. Many ate real, unprocessed food – seasonal, nutrient-dense and in harmony with their environment. As Albert Einstein once said, 'Energy cannot be destroyed; it can only transform from one form to another.'

Food, among many other things, is energy. What we consume doesn't simply disappear, it transforms into movement, vitality, and cellular repair, shaping how we think, feel and function.

Whole, natural foods contain many things our bodies need to function at their best: proteins to rebuild and repair, healthy fats for brain function, fibre to support digestion and satiety, and essential vitamins and minerals to sustain overall wellbeing. When we consume a diet consistent with our natural environment, our bodies naturally find balance – no overcomplication, diet regimes, or deprivation, just real nourishment.

For years, I've witnessed the power of whole foods to transform lives. People who thought they needed complex diet plans to feel good soon realised that the answer was much simpler – unprocess your diet and your body will do the rest. As highlighted in the research from institutions such as the World Health Organisation, The World Cancer Research Fund and The British Heart Foundation, many of today's lifestyle-related illnesses are best addressed not by adding more but by removing the excess – the artificial additives, inflammatory oils and processed sugars that disrupt our natural balance.

Nutrient-dense, whole foods can provide:

- **A Natural Compass for Health** – Whole foods work in harmony with your body's internal compass, guiding you toward satiety, true pleasure and ultimately, optimal health.
- **Sustainable, Stable Energy** – Food that supports your body, providing steady energy without extreme spikes or crashes.
- **Reduced Chronic Inflammation & Improved Digestion** – Your gut microbiome is known to thrive on diverse high-fibre wholefoods. This can lead to fewer issues with digestive problems such as constipation, bloating and discomfort. Improved gut health supports a reduction in dietary inflammation, which can help decrease long-term inflammatory health problems.
- **Healthy Weight** – Wholefoods, when eaten as part of a balanced lifestyle, can support a naturally healthy body size without deprivation and no extremes.
- **Radiant, Healthy Skin** – Your skincare starts in the kitchen. There are a number of important nutrients in wholefoods which can support and protect skin health.
- **Deep, Restful Sleep** – Nourishing your body with wholefoods can help maintain good restful sleep, supporting your body's daily recovery and meaning you wake up feeling truly recharged.
- **Balanced Overall Well-Being** – When your dietary patterns are based around whole, natural, unprocessed foods, you help to support many systems across the body, encouraging physical, mental and emotional wellbeing.

The beauty of this shift is that we don't need to retreat into the wilderness, forage for every meal, or master survival skills to reconnect with real food. The key is much simpler – learning to trust your instincts, staying open to change and equipping yourself with the right tools. And it all starts in your kitchen. By stocking it with the essentials, you create an environment where whole-food living becomes second nature.

What Makes a Food Processed?

Let's get one thing clear: not all processing is bad. Freezing berries, cooking lentils, or blending whole almonds into almond butter – these are all forms of processing. But there's a difference between what can be done in your kitchen and what happens in factories where food is broken down, stripped of its natural parts, then reassembled with synthetic additives into something far less nourishing, tasty and satisfying.

Take oats, for example. Rolled oats are minimally processed – simply steamed and flattened so that they cook faster, while keeping their fibre and nutrients intact. Compare that to what happens to make white bread. In the process of making white flour, the grain is stripped of its bran and germ – the most nutrient-dense parts – leaving behind a refined starch that's often bleached, then fortified with synthetic vitamins to make up for what's been lost. That flour is then combined with processed oils, preservatives, emulsifiers and other additives to create a product that's soft, uniform and designed for shelf life, not to sustain life. That's ultra-processed food.

So how can you tell what's OK and what's not? Just flip the package over. The front of the packaging is marketing – designed to please the eyes and encourage you to buy the product. The back is for education. That's where the truth lies. If the ingredients list reads more like a chemistry sheet than a kitchen recipe – filled with artificial flavours, synthetic preservatives, emulsifiers and stabilisers – chances are high that it has been ultra processed. However, not every unfamiliar word in an ingredients list means a food is unhealthy. Some natural preservatives and additives can sound technical too, like ascorbic acid (vitamin C), citric acid (from citrus fruit), or lecithin (from sunflower). The goal isn't to avoid every ingredient you can't pronounce, but to learn what's real, what's synthetic and what serves your body.

That's where this book comes in. The focus is on simplicity. A good indicator is whether the product is still recognisably the original whole food ingredient, just in jarred or canned form. If so, it has only been minimally processed. If you can grow it, forage for it, or make it from scratch in your kitchen, it belongs on your plate. If it's an industrial product made from refined ingredients and synthetic additives, it's probably time to let it go. You won't find fizzy drink springs bubbling out of the earth, or candy bar trees growing in your local forest.

That said, we live in the real world and convenience matters. Tinned lentils, jarred tomatoes, frozen spinach – these are all an important part of a practical whole-food kitchen. Just check the label and skip anything packed with junk. (See What to Remove From Your Kitchen on page 21 for a full breakdown.)

This isn't about restriction, it's about re-education. Over time, your tastebuds will recalibrate, your body will find balance and the desire for fake foods will fade. Whole-food living isn't a diet. It's a return to what's real.

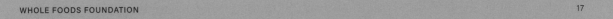

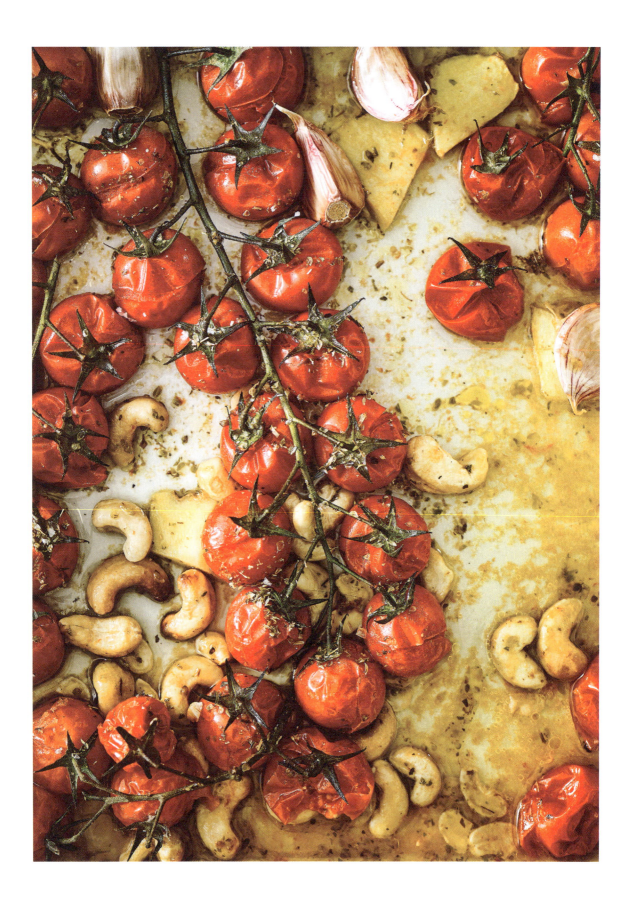

ESSENTIAL INGREDIENTS

Humans naturally look for the path of least resistance. However, in today's world, that often means fast food – cheap, effortless and instantly gratifying. A drive-thru meal takes minutes, while preparing fresh, whole food requires time, effort and intention.

But convenience shouldn't come at the cost of health and happiness. If we want to thrive, we need to create an environment where making the right choice is the easy choice. That starts in the kitchen. The best way to set yourself up for success is to remove processed foods and replace them with whole, nutrient-dense alternatives. Stocking your space with the right ingredients makes eating whole, natural foods effortless, shifting healthy eating from something that feels like work to something that feels natural.

Some of these foods might be new to you. Some might already be staples in your kitchen. You don't need access to every single one of them right away. It's about expanding your options, not limiting them.

Many people think eating whole foods means eating less variety, but the truth is, it opens up a world of abundance. Look through this list and focus on what you already know. Then, one by one, start exploring new ingredients. Maybe you swap white rice for quinoa, white flour for spelt or buckwheat flour, or you replace refined sugar with date syrup. Over time, your kitchen, and your meals, will evolve naturally.

This list is not exhaustive. There are thousands of edible fruits, vegetables, nuts, legumes, seeds, and ancient grains that have nourished people for generations. Think of this as a foundation – a reference you can return to when restocking your kitchen, building meals, or simply reminding yourself of the endless variety nature provides.

Pantry Staples:
The Foundations of a Whole-Food Kitchen

These are some of the ingredients you'll reach for time and time again to create nourishing meals effortlessly.

- **Whole Grains & Ancient Grains:** Amaranth / barley / brown rice / buckwheat / bulgur / einkorn / farro / fonio / freekeh / kamut / millet / oats / quinoa / rye / sorghum / spelt / teff / wild rice.
- **Flours:** Buckwheat flour / chestnut flour / chickpea (gram) flour / coconut flour / quinoa flour / rye flour / spelt flour / teff flour.
- **Legumes & Beans:** Black beans / black-eyed peas / butter beans (lima beans) / cannellini beans / chickpeas / kidney beans / lentils / mung beans / pigeon peas / soybeans.

- **Nuts & Seeds:** Almonds / Brazil nuts / cashews / chestnuts / chia seeds / flaxseeds / hemp seeds / macadamia nuts / pine nuts / pistachios / pumpkin seeds / sesame seeds (tahini) / walnuts / watermelon seeds.
- **Healthy Fats:** Avocados / avocado oil / extra-virgin olive oil / flaxseed oil.
- **Natural Sweeteners:** Date sugar / date syrup / honey / pure maple syrup.
- **Fermented Foods:** Kimchi / miso / raw apple cider vinegar / sauerkraut / tempeh.
- **Seaweed & Mineral-Rich Additions:** Bladderwrack / dulse / Irish sea moss / kelp / nori / wakame.
- **Essential Herbs & Spices:** Allspice / anise seed / bay leaves / cardamom / cayenne pepper / cinnamon / cloves / cumin / garlic / ginger / paprika / sea salt / turmeric.
- **Medicinal Herbs: (Please do seek medical advice before taking any medicinal herbs)** Ashwagandha / batana / black seed / bladderwrack / blessed thistle / blue vervain / burdock root / cascara sagrada / damiana / elderberry / ginseng / hops / Irish sea moss / lavender / maca / moringa / nettle / nopal / red clover / rhubarb root / sage / sarsaparilla / shea butter / valerian / yellow dock.

Fresh Produce:
What to Prioritise

Seasonal, organic and nutrient-dense produce should form the foundation of your meals.

- **Sprouts & Microgreens:** Alfalfa sprouts / broccoli sprouts / coriander (cilantro) microgreens, pea shoots, radish sprouts / sunflower sprouts / wheatgrass.
- **Leafy Greens:** Amaranth greens / bok choy / coriander / dandelion greens / kale / lettuce / parsley / purslane / Swiss chard / turnip greens / watercress / wild rocket (arugula).
- **Other Vegetables:** Asparagus / aubergine (eggplant) / broccoli / beetroot (beets) / cauliflower / carrots / daikon radish / fennel / horseradish / Jerusalem artichokes / leeks / mushrooms / nopales / okra / olives / onions / potatoes / sweet potatoes / turnips.
- **Fruits:** Apples / avocados / baobab fruit / bell peppers / berries / black sapote / camu camu / cantaloupe / chayote / cherries / coconuts / courgettes (zucchini) / cucumbers / currants / dates / dragon fruit / figs / grapes / jackfruit / limes / mangos / melons / mulberries / oranges / papayas / peaches / pears / plums / pomegranates / prickly pears / prunes / raisins / soursops / squashes / tamarinds / tomatoes.

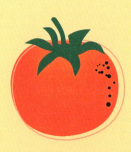
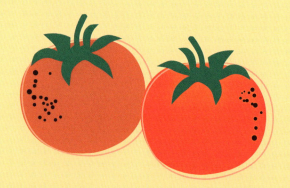

Protein Sources:
Plant-Based & High-Quality Animal Products

Protein is essential for muscle repair, energy and satiety. Whole-food protein sources include:

- **Plant-Based Proteins:** Almonds / amaranth grains / black beans / black-eyed peas / Brazil nuts / buckwheat / butter beans / cannellini beans / cashews / chestnuts / chia seeds / chickpeas / flaxseeds / hemp seeds / lentils / kidney beans / macadamia nuts / mung beans / pine nuts / pistachios / pumpkin seeds / quinoa / rye / sesame seeds (tahini) / spelt / teff / tempeh / tofu / walnuts.
- **High-Quality Animal Proteins:** Free-range eggs / goat's milk / mackerel / organic bison / organic grass-fed steak / organic Greek yogurt / wild salmon / wild sardines / tuna steak.

Building Your Whole-Food Kitchen:
What to Remove

The quality of your food doesn't just depend on what you eat, it also depends on how you prepare it. Just as processed ingredients can introduce harmful substances into your body, the wrong cookware can leach toxins into your meals, undermining the very nourishment you're striving for. Investing in safe, high-quality kitchen tools is just as important as choosing the right ingredients. Here's what to look for when building a kitchen that supports your health, not works against it.

Best Non-Toxic Cookware Options

- Cast iron
- Stainless steel
- 100% ceramic cookware
- Enamelled cast iron

Best Non-Toxic Cutting Board & Cooking Utensil Options

- Wooden cutting board & cooking utensils
- Stainless-steel utensils
- Glass cutting boards
- 100% silicone utensils

Best Non-Toxic Food Storage Container Options

- Glass containers
- Stainless steel bowls
- Silicone food bags

Best Non-Toxic Canned Food Options

- BPA-free organic canned foods
- Glass jarred versions preferable
- Cook beans, tomatoes and sauces fresh when possible

Best Non-Toxic Water Bottle Options

- Stainless steel water bottles
- Glass bottles
- High-quality water filters (i.e. Berkey)

Foraging

Foraging is a wonderful way to reconnect with nature and incorporate fresh, seasonal and nutrient-rich ingredients into your meals. It's a quiet rebellion, preserving the wisdom that has sustained us for millennia. Let's ensure this knowledge continues to thrive with us and beyond. However, it's crucial to prioritise safety and sustainability when gathering wild foods. Before foraging, please keep the following in mind:

Proper Identification

Always ensure you correctly identify plants and berries before consuming them. Some plants may look similar to others that are toxic or harmful. If you are unsure, consult an expert, use a reliable foraging guide, or attend a foraging workshop.

Harvest Responsibly

Only collect from areas where foraging is permitted and avoid plants growing near busy roads, polluted water, or areas treated with pesticides. Harvest sustainably by taking only what you need and leaving enough for wildlife and the ecosystem to thrive.

Food Safety

Wash all foraged ingredients thoroughly before using them in recipes, and follow any preparation guidelines specific to the ingredient to ensure it is safe for consumption.

Know Your Allergies

Some individuals may have allergic reactions to specific plants.
If you are foraging or eating wild foods for the first time, start with small quantities.

Legal Considerations

Familiarise yourself with local laws and regulations around foraging. Certain plants or areas may be protected and foraging may be restricted. Before foraging on private land, be sure to ask permission from the owner.

Disclaimer

The author assumes no responsibility for any harm, injury, or illness resulting from improper foraging or consumption of wild plants. Foraging is a personal responsibility and you are encouraged to educate yourself thoroughly and proceed with care.

Happy foraging and enjoy the journey of discovering the gifts of nature!

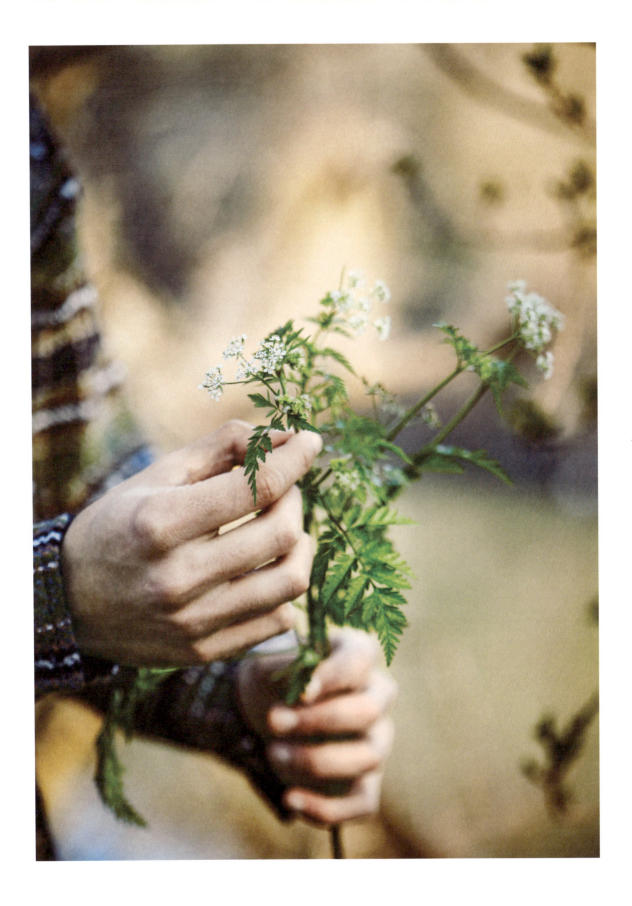

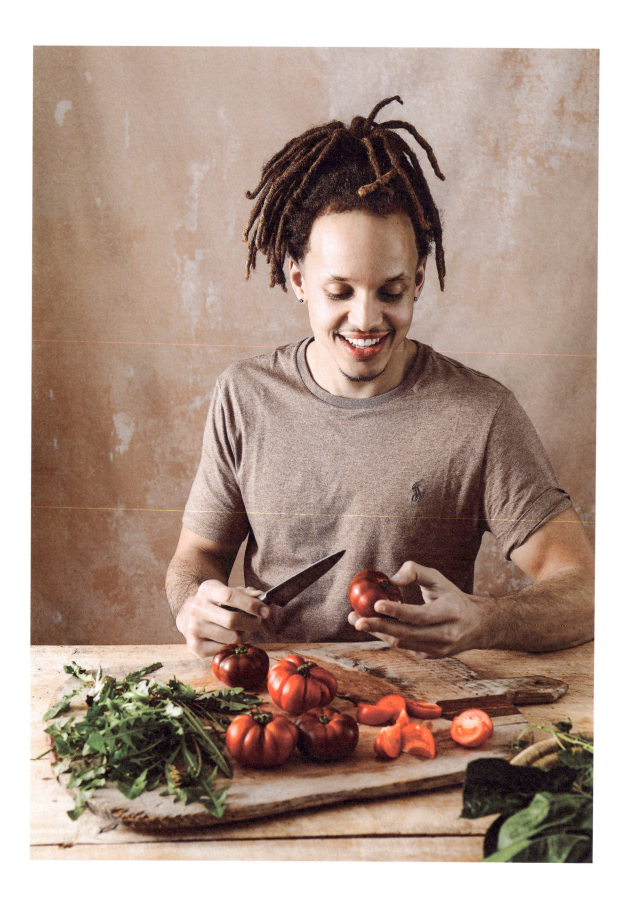

SOAKING INGREDIENTS

Why It Matters

Soaking is a simple yet powerful and ancient technique that can transform the texture, digestibility and nutritional profile of many ingredients. Whether you're working with nuts, seeds, grains, or legumes, soaking helps to remove anti-nutrients like phytic acid, reduce cooking times, and makes these ingredients easier for your body to digest and absorb.

Ingredients such as chickpeas, lentils and quinoa are nutrient powerhouses, but many of us have forgotten how to prepare them properly. This guide provides soaking times for commonly used ingredients throughout the book. Feel free to refer back to this section for a general overview whenever you're working with these ingredients.

Soaking Times for Common Ingredients

Nuts & Seeds: After soaking nuts and seeds, always rinse them thoroughly to remove any released tannins or anti-nutrients.

- **Cashews** 2–4 hours (perfect for creating creamy textures like sauces or desserts)
- **Almonds** 8–12 hours (softens them for blending or eating raw)
- **Walnuts** 4–6 hours (removes bitterness and enhances flavour)
- **Hemp seeds** 2–4 hours

Legumes: For legumes, discard the soaking water and rinse well before cooking to remove any compounds that can cause bloating.

- **Dried lentils (green, brown, red)** 4–6 hours or overnight (reduces cooking time and aids digestion)
- **Dried chickpeas** 8–12 hours (softens for cooking or blending into recipes like hummus)
- **Dried black beans** 8–12 hours (essential for even cooking and digestibility)

Grains: Soaking grains can reduce cooking time while preserving their nutrients.

- **Quinoa** 30–60 minutes (removes bitterness from saponins)
- **Rice (brown)** 6–8 hours (improves texture and reduces cooking time)
- **Rice (white)** 15–30 minutes (improves texture and reduces cooking time)
- **Oats (steel-cut or rolled)** 4–6 hours (for a creamier porridge)

HOW THE CHALLENGE WORKS

This meal plan is a guide, not a rigid rulebook. Don't feel obligated to follow its structure to the letter. The recipes in this book have been carefully selected to give you the best possible foundation, but how you implement them is entirely up to you. If you prefer to skip breakfast some mornings and focus on lunch, dinner and a snack instead, that's absolutely fine. The key issue is to listen to your body and find a rhythm that feels natural.

Repetition can be your greatest ally. If you find a meal that works for you – one that leaves you feeling satisfied and energised – there's no need to reinvent the wheel every day. For example, if you love the Quinoa Porridge, you can have it for breakfast all week in Week 1. Then, in Week 2, switch it up with the Green Goodness Smoothie to introduce a wider variety of nutrients and flavours. The goal isn't constant variety for the sake of it, but rather creating a sustainable approach that works with your lifestyle, while ensuring a diverse intake of nutrients over time.

Stay flexible, stay consistent and, most importantly, enjoy the process. The only rules?

- **Whole Ingredients Only** – Fresh fruits and vegetables, whole/ancient grains, legumes, nuts, seeds, and high-quality animal products (if you choose to include them).
- **No Refined Sugars, Additives, or Ultra-Processed Foods** – If it is not listed in the 'Essential Ingredients' section, can't be found in nature or is made up of ingredients that don't exist in their whole form, it's likely not part of this challenge.
- **Simple, Nourishing Meals** – Nothing complicated, just natural food that fuels you.
- **Listen to your Body** – No portion control or calorie counting, just eating in alignment with your hunger and satiety.

The rules are simple, but the impact is profound.

Remember, this isn't about perfection. If you slip up, you don't 'start over' – just keep moving forward. The goal is progress, not to conform to rigid rules.

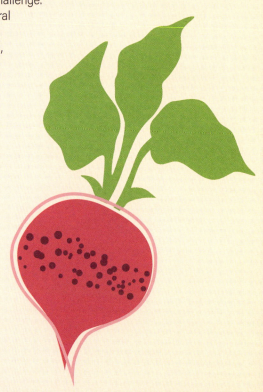

What to Expect

Week 1: Reset

The first few days may feel like a recalibration. Your body is adjusting, your tastebuds are waking up and cravings may try to pull you back into old habits. This is where most people give up – but if you push through, everything starts to shift.

Week 2: Reconnection

Your energy begins to stabilise, digestion may improve and it may feel as if your senses have sharpened. Food starts to taste different – not because anything has changed but because, for the first time in a long time, your tastebuds aren't overstimulated by artificial flavours. You begin to experience the natural sweetness of fruit, the depth of whole grains and the richness of real ingredients as they are.

Week 3: Strength

By now, your body is thriving. Your sleep may feel deeper and you should feel continued disgestion improvements. Beyond that, something deeper shifts – the way you *see* food changes. What once felt like sacrifice now feels like liberation. You're no longer drawn to foods that leave you sluggish and depleted. Your body has learned what real nourishment feels like, and it's leaning into it.

Week 4: Integration

This is where everything clicks. What started as a challenge has become second nature. Your cravings have changed and you know what makes you feel good. There's no longer a sense of restriction, just a deep understanding of what your body needs and how to honour it. This is no longer about a 30-day reset. This is about a way of living that makes you feel alive.

Unprocess is about far more than just food. It's about breaking free from the cycle of quick fixes, and rediscovering the body's self-regulating mechanism that directs us towards health and true pleasure. It's about reclaiming the power of food to support health and wellbeing, as fuel and as a source of deep nourishment.

So, whether you're here to reset, to heal, or simply to explore a new way of eating, know this: you are in control. You are the architect of your own wellbeing. You are capable. And by the end of these 30 days, you will feel a difference.

Let's get started.

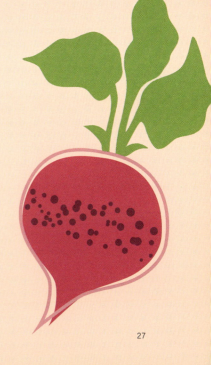

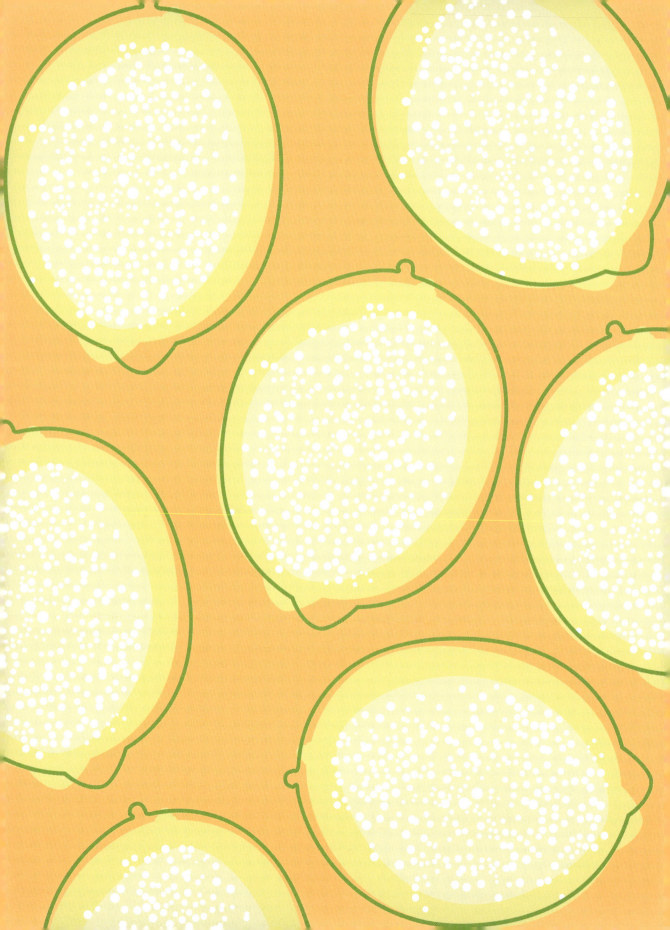

ENERGY BOOSTING
BREAKFASTS

RISE

Green Goodness Smoothie

Serves 1
Prep 2 minutes

I feel my best – physically, mentally and spiritually – when I eat a generous amount of fresh, organic leafy greens daily. My skin thanks me and, on a deeper level, they help me feel grounded and connected to the land. Yet, we rarely eat as many bitter leafy greens as our bodies crave. They are among the most abundant food sources in the world and, traditionally, we would have consumed them daily. However, modern processed foods have dulled our taste buds, making us less receptive to the natural bitterness of these essential foods. This smoothie recipe is a simple and delicious way to start your morning with a nourishing boost of fresh greens.

200ml (7fl oz/scant 1 cup)
    coconut milk
50g (1¾oz) fresh spinach
2 tbsp shelled hemp seeds
2 tbsp cashews, soaked for 2–4 hours,
    then drained (see page 25)
½ avocado
150g (5½oz) frozen mango

In a high-speed blender or food processor, combine all the ingredients and blend on high for 60–90 seconds, or until the mixture is smooth and creamy.

Pour the smoothie into a glass and enjoy immediately.

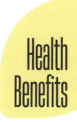

Health Benefits

This smoothie is a good source of protein and important nutrients such as folic acid and magnesium, making it a great breakfast smoothie or post-workout fuel.

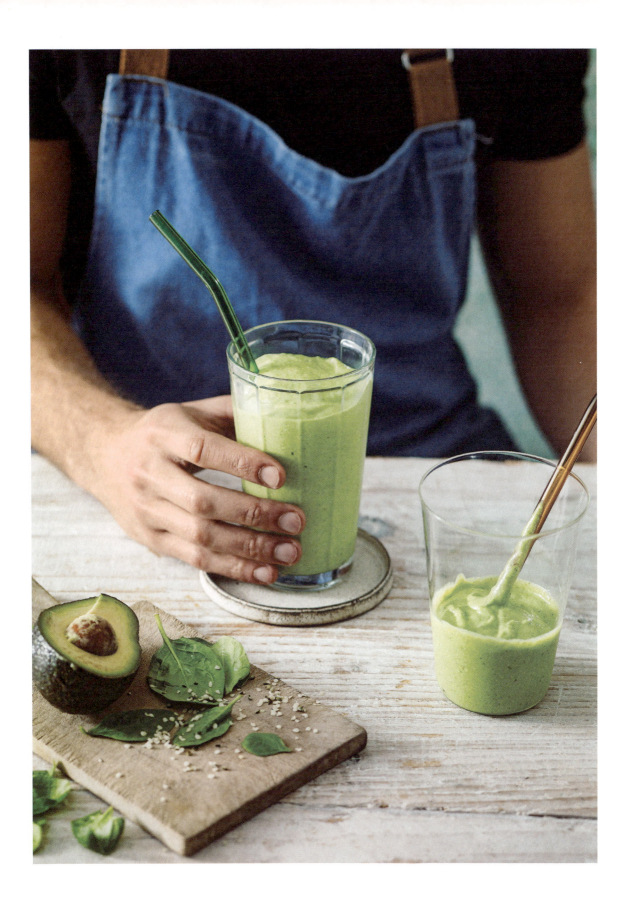

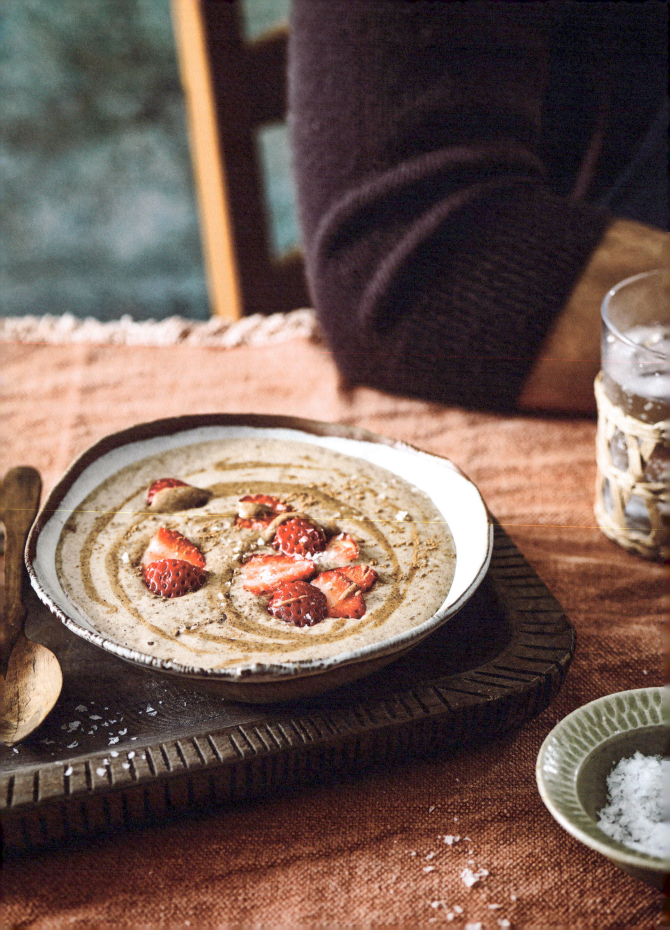

Salted Caramel Smoothie Bowl

Serves 1
Prep 10 minutes

'Salted caramel, but make it fuel.' This bowl hits all the right notes – sweet, creamy and just the right amount of salty – but without the sugar crash. Medjool dates and bananas bring that natural caramel richness, while tahini or almond butter add depth and healthy fats to keep you going. Cinnamon ties it all together with a warm, spiced kick. The best part? Every ingredient is here to work for you. Whether you need a morning boost, a post-workout recovery, or just something to satisfy those sweet cravings – this is indulgence done right.

In a high-speed blender or food processor, combine all the ingredients and blend on high until completely smooth and creamy. Adjust as needed – if you prefer a thinner consistency, add a splash more milk. For a thicker texture, let it sit in the fridge for 5–10 minutes to thicken naturally.

Pour into a bowl or glass and top with your choice of bananas, cashews, cacao nibs, a drizzle of almond butter, sesame seeds and, strawberries.

2 frozen bananas
3 medjool dates, pitted
230ml (8fl oz/1 cup) unsweetened milk of choice (coconut or almond work well)
3 tbsp tahini or almond butter
2 tbsp ground linseed (flaxseed)
1 tsp ground cinnamon
1 tsp vanilla extract
Pinch of sea salt

Toppings (optional)

Sliced bananas
Crushed cashews
Raw cacao nibs
Almond butter
Sesame seeds
Halved strawberries

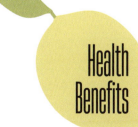

Health Benefits

Dates and bananas pack in fibre, potassium and energy-boosting carbs. Tahini or almond butter adds healthy fats to keep you satisfied. Linseeds can help maintain blood cholesterol levels. Cinnamon may help keep blood sugar stable too..

Green Smoothie Bowl

Serves 1
Prep 5 minutes

I struggled a lot with breakouts, acne and acne scars during puberty, just like many teenagers. I tried every skincare routine my sister or GP recommended. While they helped temporarily to reduce blemishes and scars, they felt more like surface-level cover-ups rather than solutions to the root cause. One of the reasons I'm so convinced of the power of the right food choices is because, after switching to a whole-foods-based diet, I started receiving compliments on my skin – something I had never experienced before. Today, after years of eating whole foods, my skin looks and feels the best it ever has. This smoothie bowl is one of my favourites and it helped me get there.

In a high-speed blender or food processor, combine all the ingredients and blend for 60–90 seconds, or until the mixture is smooth and creamy. If the mixture is too thick, add 1–2 tablespoons of coconut or almond milk.

Transfer the smoothie mixture to a bowl, and top with fruits, edible flowers, seeds and nuts of your choice.

150g (5½oz) frozen mango

40g (1½oz) kale, stalks removed and leaves chopped

3–4 medjool dates, pitted

2 frozen bananas

1 avocado (about 150g/5½oz prepared weight)

2 tbsp tahini

60g (2¼oz) Brazil nuts or cashews, soaked for 2–4 hours, then drained (see page 25, optional)

1–2 tbsp coconut or almond milk, if needed

Toppings (optional)
Sliced fresh fruit
Edible flowers
Seeds
Crushed nuts

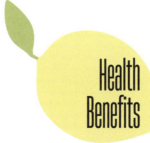

Health Benefits

This smoothie bowl contains antioxidants such as vitamin C, which support maintenance of healthy skin. Antioxidants play a really important role in protecting our body against oxidative stress, known as free radical damage.

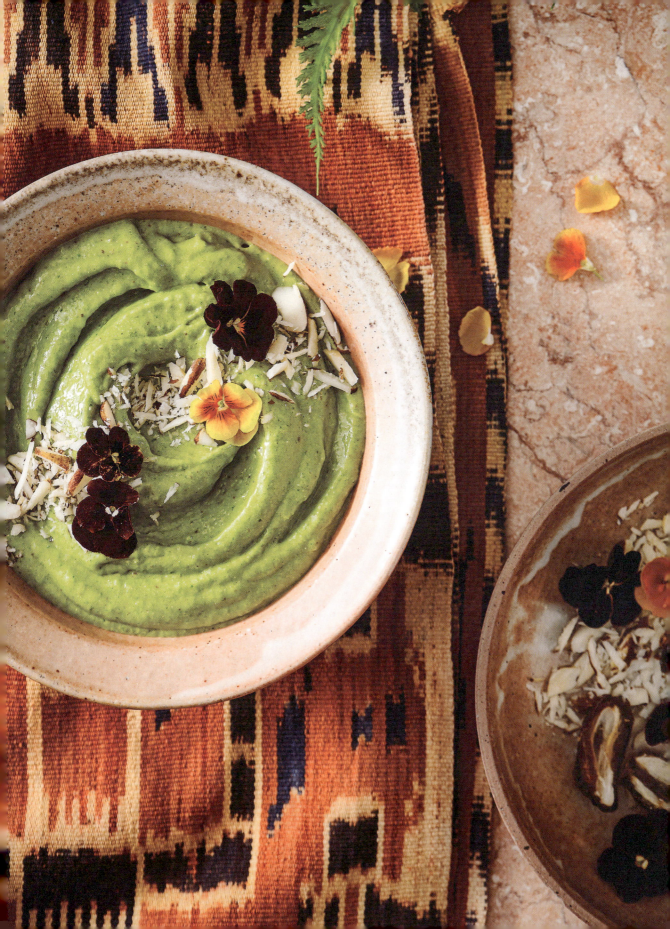

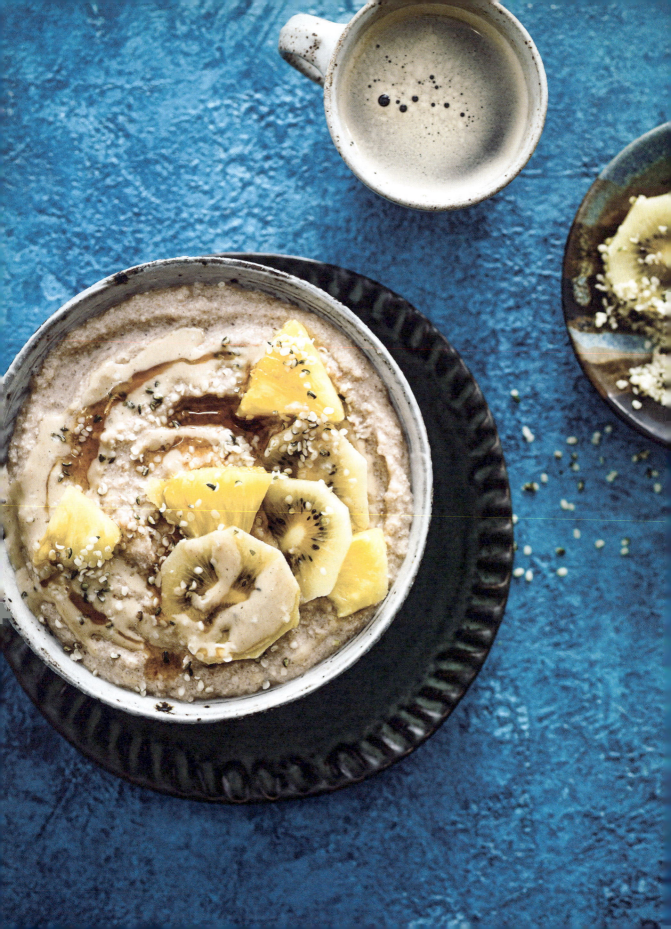

Creamy Power Porridge

A complete breakfast, for me, has four essentials: healthy fats, protein, fibre-rich carbs and vibrant fruits or veg. This Power Porridge checks all these boxes. Healthy fats come from the nuts and coconut cream, protein from the ancient grains and nuts, and fibre-rich carbs from the grains and fruits, with colourful fruit for extra goodness. Blend it all up and you have an elite breakfast to power you through the day.

Rinse the quinoa or amaranth thoroughly under cold water using a fine-mesh sieve until the water runs clear.

Place your choice of grain in a pot with 240ml (9fl oz/1 cup) water for quinoa, or 200ml (7fl oz/scant 1 cup) water for amaranth. Bring to a boil, then reduce to a simmer. Cover with a lid and cook quinoa for 10–15 minutes, or until the water is fully absorbed, or amaranth for 20–25 minutes, stirring occasionally, until tender.

Remove from the heat and leave to sit uncovered for 5–10 minutes.

Transfer the cooked grains to a blender. Add the milk, dates, banana, walnuts, ground cloves, cinnamon and creamed coconut. Blend on high until smooth and creamy. Adjust the consistency with a little more milk, if needed.

Pour the blended mixture back into the pot and warm over a low heat, stirring frequently, for 5–7 minutes, until heated through.

Serve the porridge in bowls with your favourite toppings – fresh fruit, hemp seeds, nut butter or a drizzle of tahini.

80g (2¾oz) quinoa or 65g (2¼oz) amaranth, rinsed
200ml (7fl oz/scant 1 cup) milk of choice (almond or coconut work well)
2–3 medjool dates, pitted
1 ripe banana
15–20g (½-¾oz) walnuts, chopped
¼ tsp ground cloves
1 tsp ground cinnamon
2 tbsp creamed coconut

Toppings (optional)
Fresh fruit of your choice
Shelled hemp seeds
Nut butter or tahini

Note
For improved digestibility and nutrient absorption, soak the quinoa or amaranth overnight in water before cooking (see page 25). This helps reduce its phytic acid content. Phytic acid is a natural compound that can interfere with the absorption of certain minerals. After soaking, rinse the quinoa or amaranth thoroughly.

Quinoa Porridge

Maintaining a healthy weight with unprocessed foods often means swapping common ingredients for more nutrient-dense options, such as quinoa (a complete protein and ancient grain) instead of oats. As Aris Latham said, 'There's a limited capacity to how much I can eat in a day, and I want it to count. I want to live in an expensive body!' Let's make every ingredient work for us.

Rinse the quinoa in water using a fine-mesh sieve. Repeat until the water runs clear.

In a pot, combine the rinsed quinoa with 240ml (9fl oz/1 cup) water. Bring to a boil, then reduce the heat to a low simmer. Cover and cook for 10-15 minutes, or until the water is fully absorbed. Remove from heat and leave uncovered for 5–10 minutes.

Pour in enough of your milk of choice to cover the quinoa. Bring to a boil, then simmer over a low heat for 5 minutes, stirring occasionally.

Stir in the sweetener of choice, ground cloves and cinnamon, and cook for another 5 minutes, stirring occasionally. If it becomes too dry, add a little more milk.

Remove from the heat and stir in the creamed coconut. Leave to sit for 5 minutes to absorb the flavours.

Serve the quinoa porridge in a bowl with your favourite toppings – berries, coconut flakes, hemp seeds and a drizzle of tahini. Enjoy!

80g (2¾oz) quinoa
180–240ml (6–9fl oz/¾–1 cup) plant-based milk of choice (oat, almond or coconut work well)
1 tbsp sweetener of choice (i.e. agave syrup)
¼ tsp ground cloves
1 tsp ground cinnamon
2–3 tbsp creamed coconut

Toppings (optional)
Fresh berries
Coconut flakes
Shelled hemp seeds
Tahini

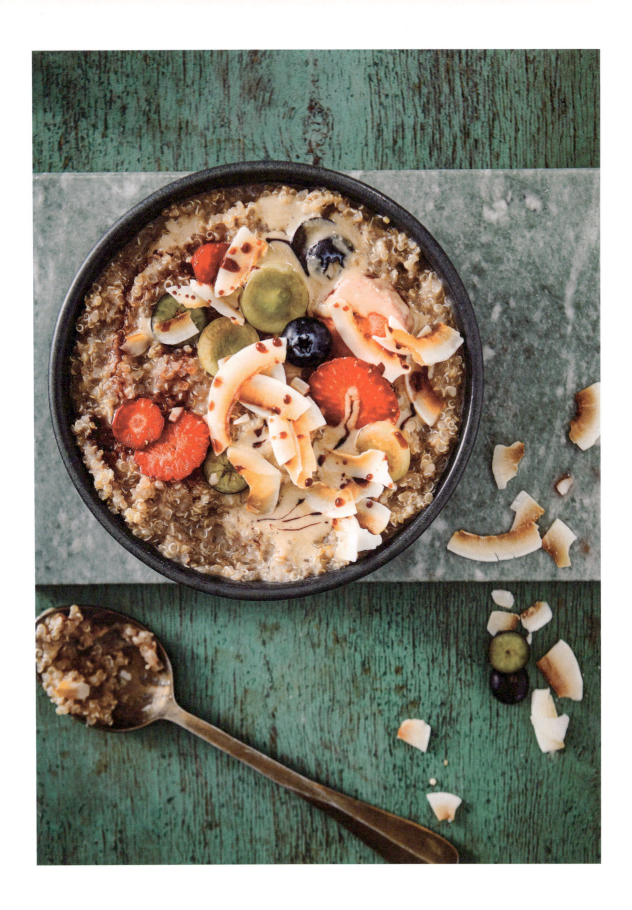

Deep Comfort Cacao Porridge

'What you seek is seeking you,' as Rumi said. Just like life, food has a way of giving you exactly what you need. Some foods cool, some energise, and some deeply ground you. This cacao porridge is all about warmth – both in flavour and function. Cacao has long been considered a sacred food, used in ancient rituals for its heart-opening, mood-lifting properties. When paired with warming spices, such as cinnamon and cloves, it creates the kind of comfort that goes beyond just taste – it's nourishment for the body and spirit. This bowl is for slow mornings, for grounding yourself before a busy day, and for those moments when you need something simple yet deeply satisfying. Five minutes, a handful of ingredients and a bowl of pure, rich goodness.

To a small saucepan, add the oats, cacao powder, cinnamon, cloves and a pinch of salt. Mix well to distribute the spices evenly. Pour in the milk and place the saucepan over a low heat. Cook gently for about 3–5 minutes, stirring continuously to prevent sticking, until the oats soften and the porridge thickens. Adjust the texture according to your preference. If you like a thicker porridge, simmer for an extra minute; if it's too thick, stir in a splash more milk.

Remove from the heat and mix in the almond butter and date syrup, letting them melt into the oats. Stir in the coconut cream at this stage, if using, for extra richness.

Spoon the porridge into a bowl and serve immediately, sprinkled with hemp seeds, pumpkin seeds, desiccated coconut and a drizzle of tahini. Enjoy warm, letting the deep flavours of cacao and warming spices do their magic.

80g (2¾oz/scant 1 cup) oats
   (or cooked quinoa or amaranth)
1 heaped tsp raw cacao powder
1 tsp ground cinnamon
½ tsp ground cloves
Pinch of sea salt
200ml (7fl oz/scant 1 cup)
   unsweetened milk of choice
   (coconut or almond work well)
1 tbsp almond butter
1 tbsp date syrup or 1 tsp maple syrup,
   to taste
2 tbsp coconut cream (optional)

Toppings (optional)
Shelled hemp seeds
Pumpkin seeds
Desiccated (dried shredded) coconut
Tahini

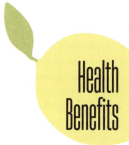

Health Benefits

Cacao is a good source of polyphenols. These are bioactive compounds that have been proven to help guard against damage caused by free radicals. It is also rich in minerals such as magnesium, potassium, iron, zinc and selenium. But not all cacao is created equal – raw cacao is the least processed and retains the most nutrients, making it the best choice for a truly nourishing bowl. Oats bring sustained energy and gut-friendly fibre, but for an even more nutrient-dense version, you can swap them for cooked ancient grains, such as quinoa, amaranth, teff or buckwheat.

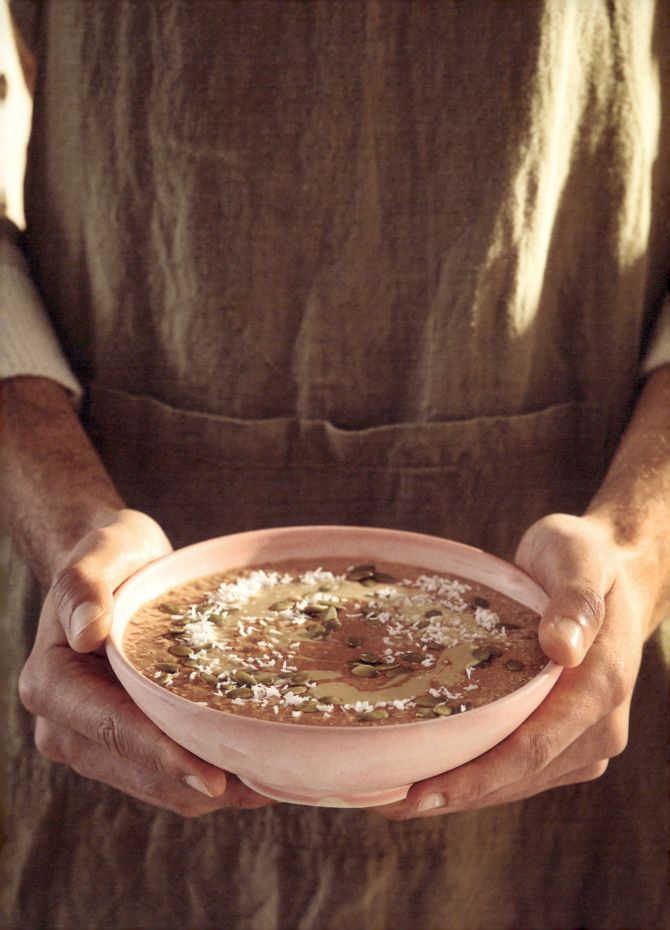

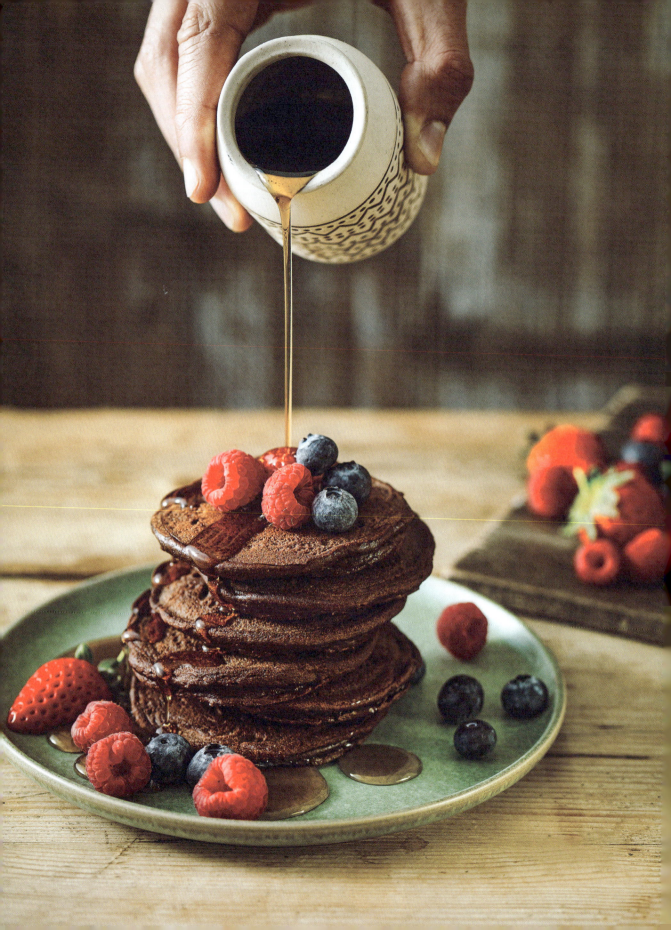

Chocolate Chickpea Pancakes

The perfect Sunday morning for me starts with pancakes. So, I had to figure out how to make pancakes that don't just taste good, but also offer nutritional value. The solution? Chickpea (or gram) flour. It doesn't just up the protein levels, making these protein pancakes without the use of nasty protein powder, but it also makes them naturally gluten-free and rich in fibre. Of course, it brings its own flavour, but in combination with the aromatic cacao, cinnamon and maple syrup, it fits very well. You can use spelt, teff, buckwheat or any other flour, in the place of chickpea flour.

In a large mixing bowl, combine the chickpea flour, cacao powder, baking powder, a pinch of salt and the maple syrup. Give it a good whisk to distribute everything evenly.

Pour in the milk and mashed banana, stirring until the batter is smooth and thick. If it feels too thick, add a splash more milk; if too thin, sprinkle in a little more flour.

Place a frying pan over a medium heat and melt a teaspoon of coconut oil to coat the surface.

Spoon in the batter, about 1 heaped or 2 regular tablespoons per pancake, giving them a little space to spread. Cook for about 3 minutes, or until the edges start to look firm and small bubbles appear on the surface.

Flip carefully and cook for another 2–3 minutes, until both sides are set and the pancakes have a soft, fluffy texture. Repeat with the rest of the batter, adding more oil as needed.

Stack the pancakes up and serve with your choice of fresh berries, crushed walnuts, a drizzle of almond butter, or more maple syrup.

150g (5½oz/1¼ cups) chickpea/gram flour (or any other flour)
60g (2¼oz) raw cacao powder
1½ tsp baking powder
Pinch of sea salt
3–4 tbsp maple syrup, plus extra for drizzling
1 ripe banana, mashed
200ml (7fl oz/scant 1 cup) unsweetened milk of choice (almond or coconut work well)
2 tbsp coconut oil

Toppings (optional)
Fresh berries
Crushed walnuts
Almond butter
Fresh berries

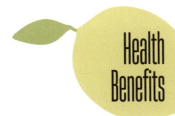

Health Benefits

Chickpea flour is a nutrient-dense flour that is also naturally gluten-free. It's rich in protein, fibre and a good source of healthy mono and polyunsaturated fats. That's why it's my go-to – nutritionally solid, easy to work with and far more affordable than most processed, gluten-free alternatives.

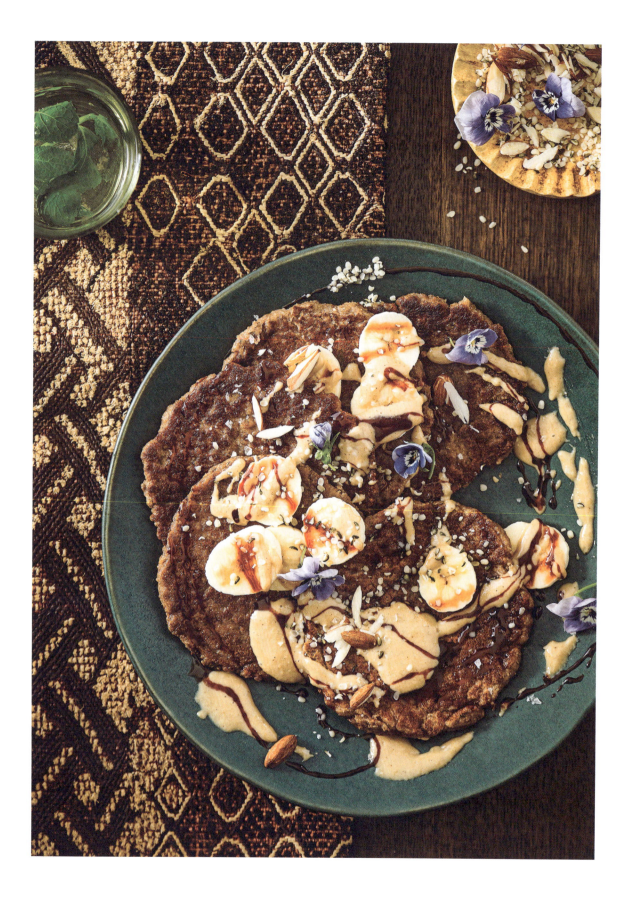

Gut—Friendly Pancakes

Serves 1–2
Prep 7 minutes
Cook 16 minutes

It's not just what you eat, it's what your body can absorb. These pancakes are built for easy digestion and maximum nourishment. Designed with digestion in mind, they skip the usual gluten and binders in favour of whole, nutrient-packed ingredients that your body can actually use. If you don't have oat flour to hand, you can easily make your own by blending oats into a fine powder.

Mix the oat flour, ground almonds, cinnamon, cloves, a pinch of salt and the chia seeds in a bowl. Stir well.

In a separate bowl, combine the mashed bananas, milk and maple syrup. Pour this mixture into the dry ingredients and mix until you have a thick pancake batter.

Place a teaspoon of coconut oil in a frying pan over a medium heat. Once hot, spoon in the batter, about a heaped tablespoon per pancake. Cook for 3–4 minutes, until bubbles form on the surface and the edges firm up, then flip and cook for another minute or so, until golden brown on both sides. Continue with the rest of the batter, adding more coconut oil to the pan, as needed.

Pile them up on plates and top with banana slices, almond butter, hemp seeds and a drizzle of date syrup, or whatever fuels your day best.

100g (3½oz/1 cup) oats, blended into a fine flour (or use store-bought oat flour)
90g (3¼oz/¾ cup) ground almonds
1 tsp ground cinnamon
½ tsp ground cloves
Pinch of sea salt
2 tbsp chia seeds
2 very ripe bananas, mashed
220ml (8fl oz/1 cup) unsweetened milk of choice (coconut or almond work well)
1–2 tbsp maple syrup (to taste)
2 tbsp coconut oil

Toppings (optional)
Sliced banana
Almond butter
Shelled hemp seeds
Date syrup

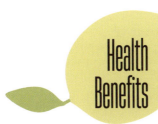

Health Benefits

Unlike most pancakes that rely on processed flour, these use ground almonds and oat flour for a boost of plant protein, fibre and minerals. The chia seeds help bind everything together while also delivering omega-3, and the bananas provide natural sweetness without refined sugar. The combination of slow-burning carbs, healthy fats and essential nutrients makes this the perfect meal to keep you fuelled, satisfied and feeling good long after breakfast is over.

Tofu Scramble

This was one of the first recipes I created when I embraced a plant-centred lifestyle. To this day, it's still a top recommendation for anyone transitioning intentionally to eating more plants. The tofu provides a sense of completeness, with a texture and consistency that feel familiar to those accustomed to animal-based foods. It's a comforting and satisfying dish that makes the shift feel less extreme.

Drain the tofu and pat it dry with a paper towel. Using a fork or your hands, crumble the tofu into chunks resembling scrambled eggs.

In a bowl, whisk together the turmeric, onion powder, garlic powder, tahini and kala namak or sea salt, if using. Gradually stir in the almond or coconut milk until the mixture is smooth and well combined.

Heat the olive oil in a pan over a medium-high heat. Add the crumbled tofu and cook for 5–7 minutes, stirring occasionally, until lightly browned.

Pour the spice sauce over the tofu and stir to coat evenly. Cook for 1–2 minutes, allowing the flavours to meld and the sauce to thicken slightly.

Spoon the scrambled tofu onto the sourdough toast. Garnish with fresh chives and diced tomato, if desired.

400g (14oz) firm tofu
½ tsp ground turmeric
½ tsp onion powder
½ tsp garlic powder
2 tbsp tahini
½ tsp kala namak (black salt) or sea salt (optional)
120ml (4fl oz/½ cup) almond or coconut milk
1 tbsp extra-virgin olive oil

For Serving
1–2 slices sourdough, toasted
Handful of fresh chives, finely chopped (optional)
½ tomato, diced (optional)

Note
Kala namak, also known as black salt, adds a sulfuric, egg-like flavour to the dish and can be adjusted to taste.

Health Benefits

While turmeric enhances the dish with its vibrant, yellow colour, it also offers potential health benefits. Rich in curcumin, turmeric is known for its antioxidant and anti-inflammatory properties, which may help protect the body from certain cancers.

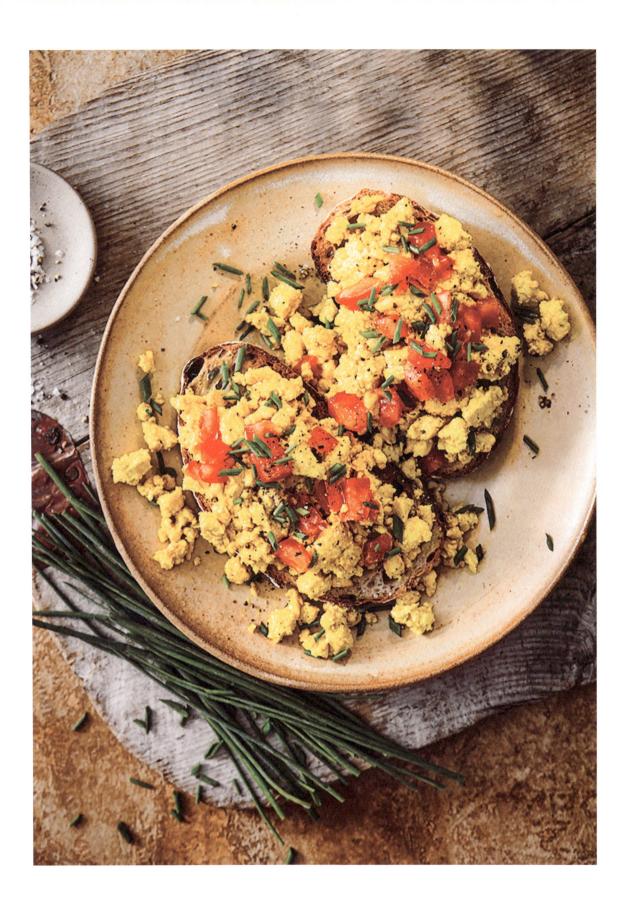

Hemp Scramble

Nutritionally, this might be the most complete alternative to scrambled eggs I've come across. I remember trying to pinpoint what makes eggs so nutritious – it's the balance of healthy fats, complete protein and essential nutrients, like zinc and B vitamins. By blending fatty milk, hemp seeds and olive oil, you achieve a similar combination of nutrients that not only mimics the nutrition of eggs but also creates an egg-like consistency. The finishing touch is the kala namak, or black salt, which adds an eggy taste that leaves even the most sceptical plant-based critics in awe. This has become my go-to Sunday morning recipe.

Add the soaked hemp seeds, turmeric, onion powder, garlic powder, kala namak or sea salt and milk to a high-speed blender or food processor. Blend until smooth, scraping down the sides to ensure a consistent texture.

Place a non-stick frying pan or stainless-steel skillet over a medium-high heat. Once hot, add the olive oil and heat until it shimmers. Pour the batter into the pan and leave to cook undisturbed for about 1 minute, until it begins to bubble.

Using a wooden spoon or silicone spatula, gently move the batter around the skillet, forming fluffy curds. Continue to cook for 1–2 minutes, stirring occasionally, until the scramble reaches your desired texture. For a softer scramble, cook for less time. For a firmer texture, cook for a little longer.

Serve warm, garnished with fresh chives, and alongside some sourdough toast and avocado, if desired.

140g (5oz) shelled hemp seeds, soaked for 2–4 hours, then drained (see page 25)
1 tsp ground turmeric
1 tsp onion powder
1 tsp garlic powder
½ tsp kala namak (black salt) or sea salt, to taste
225ml (8fl oz/scant 1 cup) unsweetened milk of choice (coconut or almond work well)
3 tbsp extra-virgin olive oil

For Serving
Handful of fresh chives, finely chopped
1–2 slices sourdough, toasted
sliced avocado (optional)

Health Benefits

Hemp seeds are a rich source of all essential amino acids, making them an excellent plant-based protein option.

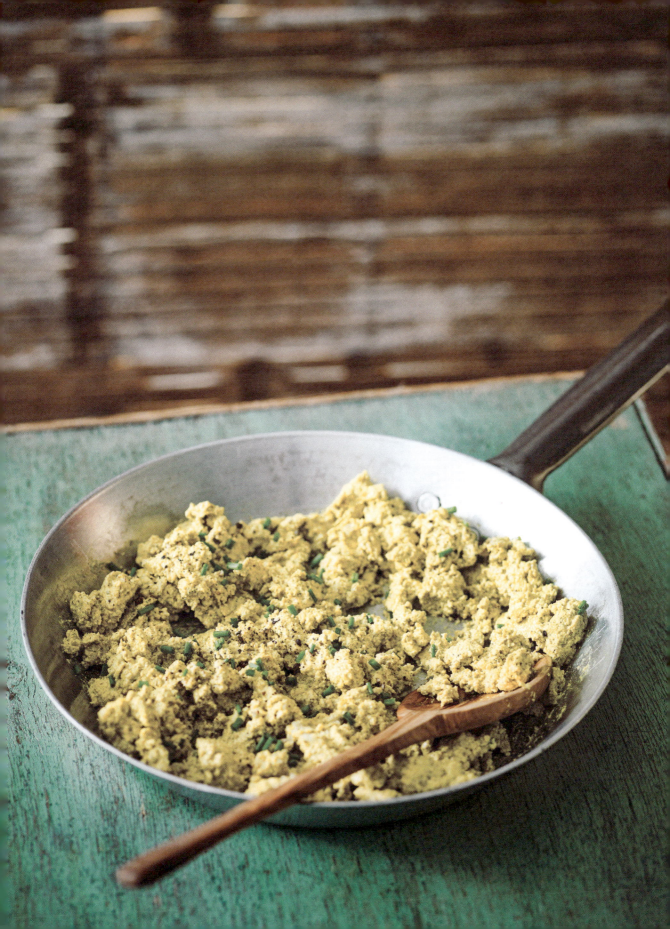

Breakfast Vitality Blend

'Every time you eat or drink, you are either feeding disease or fighting it,' as Ann Wigmore said. Food isn't just fuel, it's medicine, energy and restoration. But some days, there's no time to prep a full meal, and that's where this smoothie comes in. Quick, nourishing and packed with everything your body needs, it's the perfect fix for a rushed morning. Mango and banana bring natural sweetness, and spinach floods the body with chlorophyll and iron. But the real power here? The Brazil nuts and hemp seeds – they are tiny but support the immune system, brain function and overall vitality. Eat to thrive!

Place all the ingredients in a high-speed blender or food processor. Blend for about 30–60 seconds, until smooth, scraping down the sides if needed.

Adjust the texture, according to your preference. For a thicker smoothie, add a few ice cubes or add another frozen banana. For a thinner consistency, add a splash more coconut water.

Pour and enjoy immediately.

1 banana, fresh or frozen, plus 1 extra if needed

100g (3½oz) frozen mango

1 cube frozen spinach (or 1 handful fresh spinach)

2 tbsp shelled hemp seeds (or cashews)

2 Brazil nuts

200ml (7fl oz/scant 1 cup) unsweetened coconut water

1 tbsp chia seeds (optional)

Ice cubes, if needed

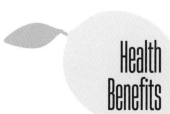

Health Benefits

This smoothie is fuel in its purest form – quick to make, easy to digest and packed with nutrients. Hemp seeds bring complete protein and essential omega-3, keeping you strong and energised, while Brazil nuts provide selenium, a key mineral for immune support and hormone balance. Spinach floods the body with chlorophyll, iron and folate, while mango and banana offer fibre, natural sweetness and steady energy. Add chia seeds for an extra omega-3 and fibre boost!

Chickpea Scramble

Chickpea flour is one of the most nutrient-dense flour options out there. Naturally gluten-free and packed with fibre and protein, it's the perfect base for this plant-based alternative to scrambled eggs. I don't think of it as a replacement but rather an exciting alternative – especially for those looking to reap the benefits of adding more plant diversity to their diet. Increased fibre intake supports digestive health and helps relieve constipation. A quick, nourishing and satisfying breakfast option!

In a medium bowl, combine the chickpea flour, milk, onion powder, garlic powder, maple syrup, turmeric and salt, if using. Whisk together until smooth and lump-free. Set aside.

Put the olive oil in a non-stick frying pan or stainless-steel skillet over a medium-high heat. Add the chopped onion and cook for 3–5 minutes, stirring occasionally, until softened.

Stir in the peppers and tomato, and sauté for 2–3 minutes, until the vegetables are tender.

Pour the chickpea batter into the pan over the sautéed vegetables. Cook undisturbed for about 2 minutes, allowing the edges to firm up. Once the batter begins to set, use a spatula to break it up into pieces, flipping and scrambling the mixture for 3–4 minutes, until fully cooked and no longer wet.

Stir in the basil and mix until evenly combined.

Transfer the scramble to a bowl and serve immediately.

60g (2¼oz/¾ cup) chickpea flour

120ml (4fl oz/½ cup) unsweetened milk of choice (coconut or almond work well)

2 tsp onion powder

1 tsp garlic powder

1 tsp maple syrup

¼ tsp ground turmeric

1 tsp sea salt (optional)

1 tsp extra-virgin olive oil

50g (1¾oz) brown onion, finely chopped

50g (1¾oz) red or yellow bell pepper, deseeded and chopped

40g (1½oz) tomato, chopped

1 handful basil, leaves finely chopped

Notes

You can include other vegetables, such as spinach or mushrooms, for extra flavour and nutrition. For a more savoury taste, replace sea salt with a pinch of kala namak (black salt).

Nature's Energy Drink

Serves 3–4
Prep 7 minutes

Before Red Bull, Powerade or Gatorade, there were fruits. Before shop-bought sweets, there were fruits. Nature set the blueprint. Our bodies have adapted to digest and process natural foods for millions of years, while modern energy drinks have only existed within our grandparents' lifetime. To truly energise your body, you need to return to the juice of fruits – the original sport drink. This is the ideal pre-workout boost, thanks to the hydrating properties of melon and the kick of ginger.

Place the watermelon chunks, ginger, lemon juice and honey, if using, in a high-speed blender or food processor. Blend for 30–60 seconds, or until the mixture is completely smooth. For a smoother texture, strain the juice through a fine-mesh sieve or cheesecloth to remove any pulp.

Pour the juice into glasses and serve immediately.

1kg (2lb 4oz) watermelon, cut into chunks (about ¼ watermelon)
Thumb-sized piece of fresh root ginger, peeled and grated
Juice of 1 lemon
1–2 tbsp raw honey (optional)

Note
Add a few fresh mint leaves to the blender for a cooling twist. The ingredients in this drink assimilate so well, you can almost instantly feel the energy boost.

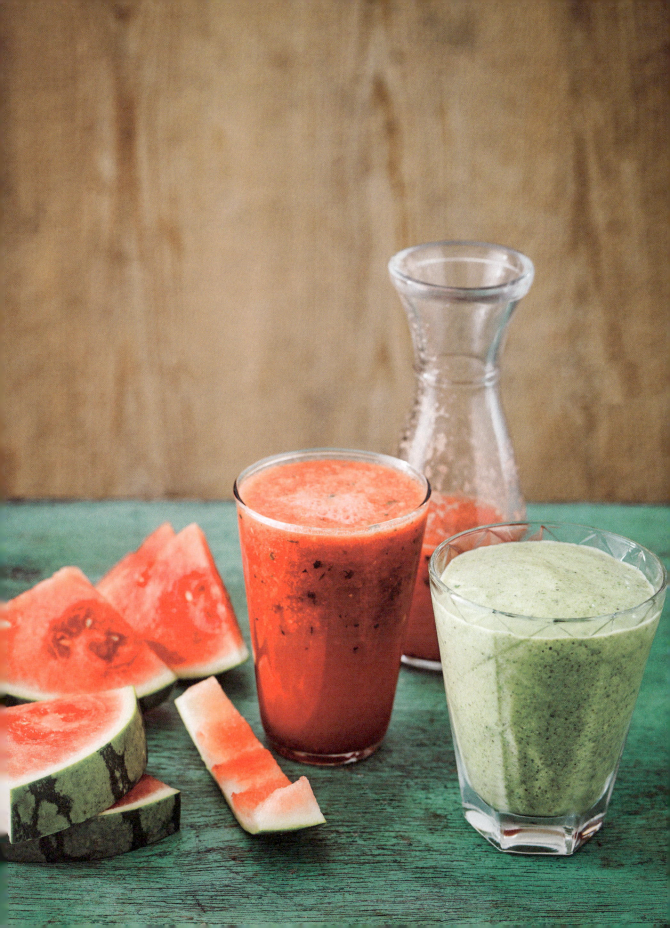

Nutty Heaven

The smoothie that dreams are made of. The natural sweetness of bananas and the caramel-like flavour of dates, combined with the nutty richness of walnuts and hemp seeds. Everything is then balanced with a touch of bitterness and warmth from cacao, cinnamon and cloves. The result is a smoothie with a consistency and taste that feels almost too good to be healthy. It's the perfect treat to start your morning or snack to power you through the day.

In a high-speed blender or food processor, combine all the ingredients and blend on high until the mixture is smooth and creamy.

Pour the smoothie into a glass and enjoy immediately.

360ml (12fl oz/1½ cups) coconut or almond milk
1 ripe banana
60g (2¼oz) walnuts
15g (½oz) shelled hemp seeds
3–4 medjool dates, pitted
2 tbsp raw cacao powder
1 tsp ground cinnamon
½ tsp ground cloves

Mango Lassi

The king of fruits – a mango is more than just a health food, it holds a deeper significance. When I think of a mango, I'm reminded of how food can impact not just the body, but the spirit. Albert Einstein said, 'Energy cannot be destroyed, it can only transform.' Thriving in the heat, a mango carries cooling energy. Eating one can help bring balance, especially in hot and stressful moments. Personally, a mango is my go-to for grounding when life feels a little too intense.

In a high-speed blender or food processor, combine all the ingredients and blend on high until the mixture is smooth and creamy.

Serve immediately – this refreshing drink is perfect for any time of day.

2 mangos (about 400g–500g/14oz–1lb 2oz combined weight), peeled and diced
120ml (4fl oz/½ cup) coconut milk
2 mint leaves
1 frozen banana
Pinch of ground cardamom or ground cinnamon

Note
Cardamom has a very strong aroma, so add it carefully. If preferred, you can replace it with nutmeg, for a milder taste.

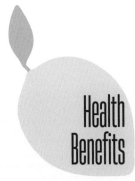

Health Benefits

Mangos have a high beta-carotene content which helps support a healthy immune system.

Liquid Gold – Turmeric Elixir

Before coffee shops there were healing tonics. For centuries people have turned to turmeric for strength, warmth and deep restoration. This isn't just a drink; it's a daily ritual, a slow fuel that works with your body, not against it. Turmeric's anti-inflammatory powers make it perfect for soothing digestion, easing aches and keeping the immune system strong. The honey rounds it out with natural sweetness and antimicrobial benefits, while the warm milk makes it comforting, grounding and exactly what you need, whether you're starting your day or winding it down. A gentle alternative to coffee, a soothing nightcap, or just a moment to pause – this is nourishment in its simplest form.

250ml (9fl oz/generous 1 cup) unsweetened milk of choice (coconut or almond work well)
1 tsp ground turmeric
1 tsp raw honey (or maple syrup)
Pinch of ground black pepper (optional)
Pinch of ground cinnamon (optional)

Heat the milk in a small pan over a low-medium heat until warm, but not boiling.

Whisk in the turmeric until fully dissolved.

Remove from the heat and leave to cool slightly before stirring in the honey. For extra depth, add a pinch of pepper to enhance turmeric absorption or a sprinkle of cinnamon for natural warmth.

Mix well and drink while it's still warm.

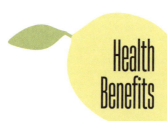

Health Benefits

Turmeric is one of the most powerful anti-inflammatory foods, known to support digestion, ease joint pain and strengthen the immune system. But here's the key – curcumin, the active compound in turmeric, needs black pepper to be properly absorbed. A pinch of black pepper boosts its bioavailability by up to 2000 per cent, making sure your body actually gets the benefits. Honey adds antioxidant and antimicrobial properties, while warm milk makes this tonic soothing and grounding.

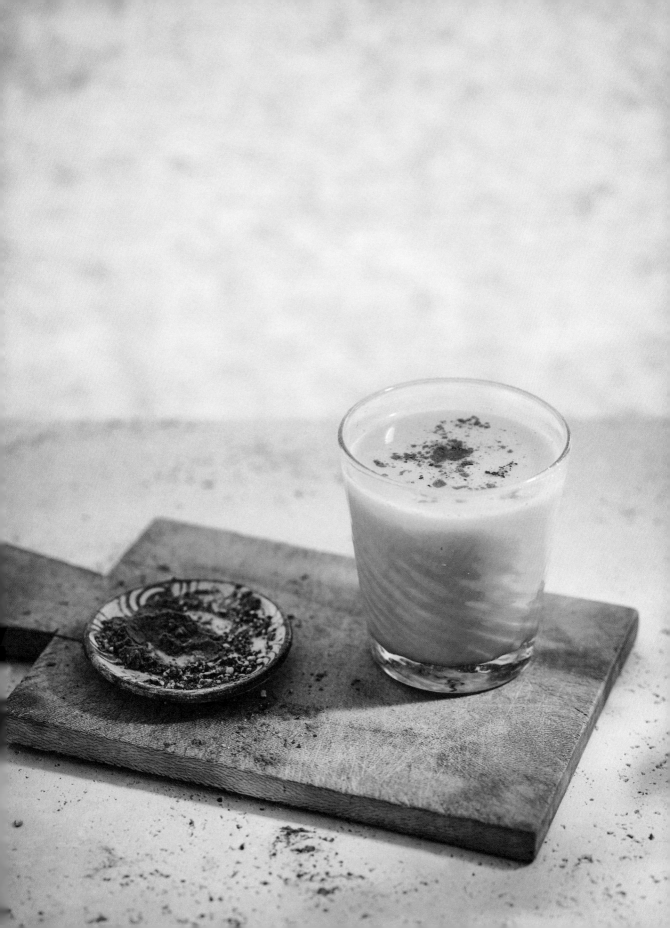

Milk Alternative

What makes milk so nourishing from a nutritional perspective? It's the combination of healthy fats, complete protein and essential nutrients, such as B vitamins and calcium. Reducing or removing dairy from your diet means finding suitable alternatives, but options like oat milk (oats and water) or soy milk (soybeans and water) often fall short in nutrient density when compared to animal-based milks. Which is why I created this alternative – it's not only delicious but also nutritionally dense. Eat to thrive!

50g (1¾oz) shelled hemp seeds
1 handful of nuts of your choice (Brazil nuts, walnuts or cashews work well)
Pinch of sea salt
3 medjool dates, pitted
½ tsp ground cinnamon (optional)
A few drops of pure vanilla extract (optional)

In a high-speed blender, combine the hemp seeds and nuts with 1 litre (35fl oz/4¼ cup) water, the salt, dates, cinnamon and vanilla extract, if using. Blend for 1–2 minutes, or until the mixture is smooth and creamy.

If a smoother texture is preferred, strain the milk through a nut-milk bag or fine mesh sieve into a jar or bowl.

Pour the milk into a glass jar and store in the fridge for up to 4 days. Shake well before serving.

Health Benefits

Hemp seeds are a rich source of complete plant-based protein, containing essential amino acids. While cow's milk has a different nutritional profile, this milk, combined with the healthy fats from the nuts, is a nutrient-dense alternative.

Creamy Weight–Gain Smoothie

Serves 1

Prep 2 minutes

Can you build muscle on a plant-centred lifestyle? How do you gain healthy weight with plant-based foods? What should you eat to fuel muscle growth? Here's the answer: the Creamy Weight Gain Smoothie. No need for protein powder – this smoothie combines healthy fats and amino-acid-rich ingredients, making it my go-to drink post-workout or whenever I want to support muscle growth naturally. Simple, effective and delicious.

In a high-speed blender or food processor, combine all the ingredients and blend on high for 60–90 seconds, or until the mixture is smooth and creamy.

Pour the smoothie into a glass and enjoy cold.

480ml (17fl oz/2 cups) coconut milk
40g (1½oz) walnuts, chopped
60g (2¼oz) tahini
3–5 medjool dates, pitted
1 avocado
2 tbsp hemp seeds

SPEEDY LUNCHES THAT FUEL

SHINE

Nourishing Broccoli Soup

When time is short but your body's calling for a reset, this soup has you covered. It's fresh, vibrant and packed with nutrients that cleanse, energise and nourish – all in under 10 minutes. Think of it as a quick reboot, a way to flood your system with greens, fibre and plant-based protein, without spending hours in the kitchen. Whether you need a light meal after a weekend of indulgence, a midweek boost, or just a simple way to eat more greens, this is the one. Quick, cleansing and effortlessly good.

Put the olive oil in a large pan over a medium heat. Add the garlic and cumin, and season with salt and pepper. Cook for 1 minute until fragrant.

Add the broccoli florets and stir well to coat in the spices. Cook for 5–6 minutes until tender.

Toss in the spinach and leave to wilt for 1–2 minutes, stirring occasionally.

Transfer everything to a high-speed blender or food processor, and add the drained beans, coriander, lemon juice and coconut milk. Blend until smooth and creamy.

Return the soup to the pan and warm over a low heat, if needed. Adjust the seasoning to taste. Serve in one or two bowls drizzled with olive oil and with more coriander sprinkled over.

1 tbsp extra-virgin olive oil, plus extra for drizzling
4 garlic cloves, minced
1 tbsp ground cumin
1 head of broccoli, broken into florets
250g (9oz) fresh spinach
1 x 400g (14oz) can butter (lima) beans, drained and rinsed (235g/8½oz drained weight)
Handful of fresh coriander (cilantro), plus extra to garnish
Juice of 1 lemon
650ml (23fl oz/2⅔ cups) coconut milk
Sea salt and black pepper

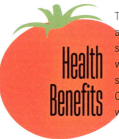

Health Benefits

This is the kind of meal that sets the tone for the week ahead or helps you reset after a long one. Light yet nourishing, it's packed with chlorophyll-rich greens that support digestion. Broccoli and spinach flood your body with fibre and antioxidants, while cannellini beans provide plant-based protein to keep you balanced and satisfied. The lemon juice not only adds a fresh, bright kick but also delivers vitamin C to maintain our immune system and enhance iron absorption. A quick, effortless way to nourish and recharge – whenever you need it most.

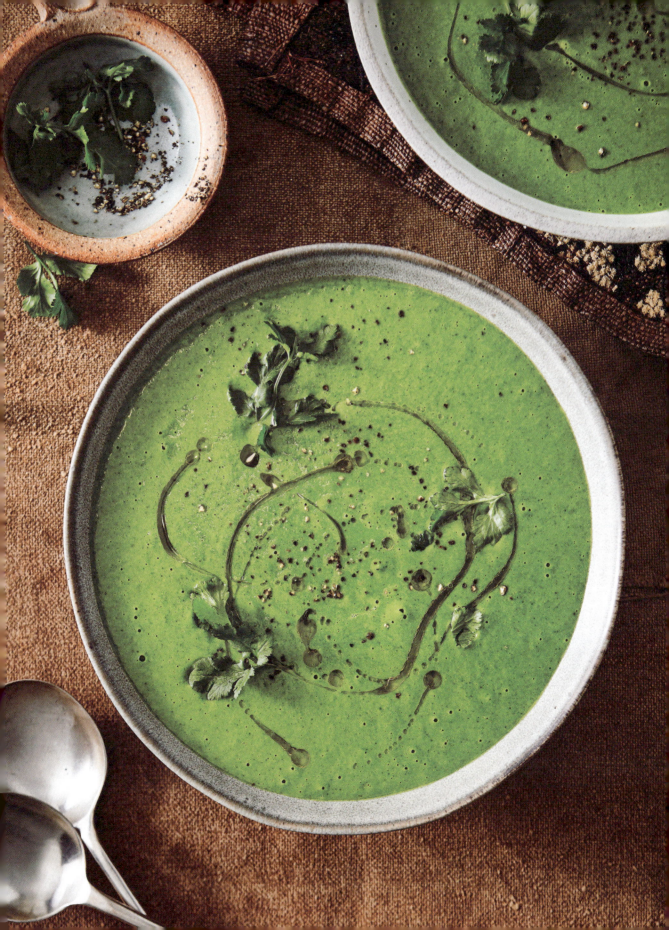

Roasted Tomato & Cashew Soup

Serves 2
Prep 15 minutes
Cook 40 minutes

Here's the secret to the best tomato soup of all time: cashews. Adding roasted cashews doesn't just make it incredibly creamy, it also boosts the protein and mineral content. With the rich creaminess of coconut milk and the natural sweetness of tomatoes, this soup is pure comfort in a bowl. Trust me, seconds are guaranteed!

Preheat the oven to Fan 160°C/180°C/350°F/Gas 4 and line a baking tray with parchment paper.

Slice the tomatoes in half and remove the stalks. Arrange them (cut sides up) with the cashews, ginger and garlic cloves on the prepared baking tray. Drizzle the olive oil over the ingredients and sprinkle with the dried oregano, salt and pepper. Roast in the preheated oven for 25–30 minutes, checking occasionally to ensure the garlic and ginger do not burn.

Remove the tray from the oven and transfer the roasted ingredients, including any juices from the tray, into a large pot. Carefully squeeze the roasted garlic out of their skins. Add the coconut milk, a handful of the basil and the cayenne pepper, and stir to combine. Place over a medium heat and bring to a boil. Reduce the heat to a simmer and cook for 10 minutes.

Using a stick blender, high-speed blender or food processor, blend the soup until smooth and creamy.

Garnish with the remaining basil leaves, a drizzle of olive oil, a sprinkle of pepper and more cayenne pepper.

1kg (2lb 4oz) tomatoes (cherry or vine tomatoes work well)
60g (2¼oz) cashews
20g (¾oz) fresh root ginger, peeled
4 garlic cloves in their skins
3 tbsp extra-virgin olive oil, plus extra for drizzling
1 tsp dried oregano
1 tsp sea salt
1 tsp ground black pepper, plus extra to garnish
500ml (17fl oz/generous 2 cups) coconut milk
2 handfuls of fresh basil
½ tsp cayenne pepper, plus extra to garnish

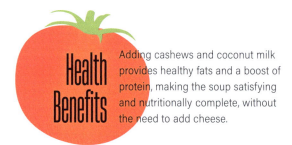

Health Benefits
Adding cashews and coconut milk provides healthy fats and a boost of protein, making the soup satisfying and nutritionally complete, without the need to add cheese.

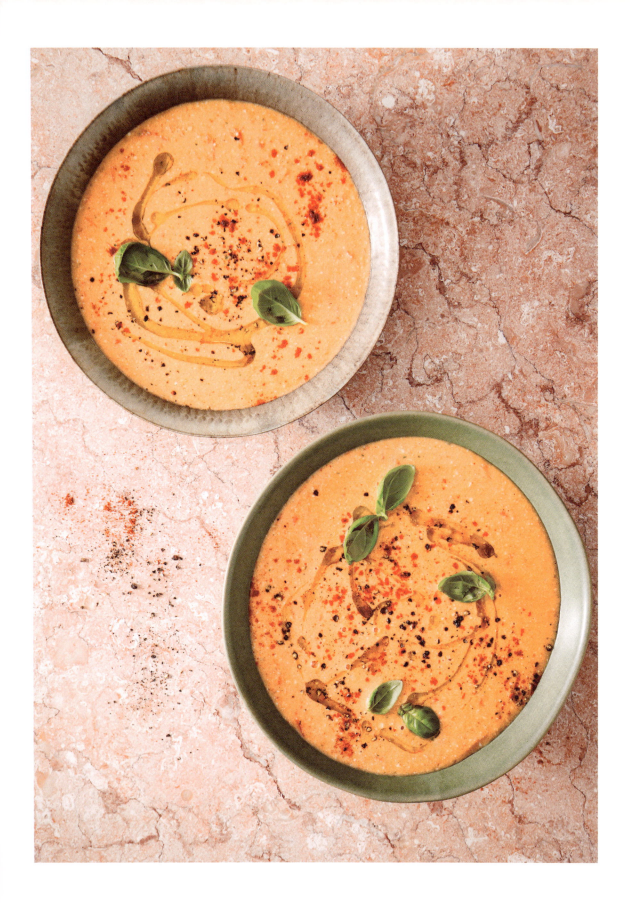

Lentil Soup

Serves 2
Prep 10 minutes
Cook 55 minutes

Growing up in the German countryside, this was one of my mum's go-to dishes. In Germany, it's often considered a 'struggle meal' because it uses simple, affordable ingredients. But for me, it's one of the most comforting and satisfying soups I've ever tasted. As soon as autumn or winter sneaks up on us, or on a rainy day, this soup is the first thing that comes to mind. It's also a great way to sneak in vegetables, like celery, making it perfect for those who aren't fans.

Heat the olive oil in a large pot over a medium heat. Add the chopped onion and minced garlic, and cook for about 2 minutes, until soft and aromatic.

Stir in the chopped carrot and celery, and cook for 7–10 minutes, stirring occasionally, until the vegetables are tender and the onion is sweet and golden.

Add the lentils, chopped tomatoes, stock, cumin, cinnamon, ground cloves, paprika and bay leaves, and stir well to combine. Increase the heat to bring the mixture to a gentle boil, then reduce the heat to medium-low, cover with a lid and simmer for 35–40 minutes, or until the lentils are tender. Stir the mixture from time to time to prevent sticking or burning.

For the best consistency, remove the bay leaves and use a stick blender to blend the soup slightly with a couple of quick pulses. If the soup is too thick, add some water. Stir in the baby spinach, if using, during the last few minutes of cooking for extra greens. Season with salt and pepper to taste and squeeze in the fresh lemon juice just before serving. Garnish with fresh coriander and serve with toasted sourdough.

2 tbsp extra-virgin olive oil

1 brown onion, chopped

2 garlic cloves, minced

1 large carrot, chopped

2 celery sticks, chopped

400g (14oz) dried brown lentils, rinsed, soaked for 4–6 hours or overnight, then drained (see page 25)

1 × 400g (14oz) can chopped tomatoes

1.5 litres (2¾ pints/6½ cups) vegetable stock

1 tsp ground cumin

1 tsp ground cinnamon

½ tsp ground cloves

1 tsp paprika

2 bay leaves

Juice of 1 lemon

Small handful of fresh coriander (cilantro), chopped

Handful of baby spinach (optional)

Sea salt and black pepper

2 slices sourdough bread, toasted, to serve

Note
Green or brown lentils work best for this recipe.

Chickpea Protein Smoothie

Frozen chickpeas are a protein-packed alternative to frozen bananas in this smoothie. Their neutral taste and creamy texture pair perfectly with the nuttiness of almond butter and hemp seeds, the natural sweetness of dates, and the warm flavours of cinnamon and cloves. It's the ultimate post-workout smoothie to support muscle growth naturally.

360ml (12fl oz/1½ cups) coconut milk
120g (4¼oz) frozen chickpeas
   (garbanzo beans)
1 tbsp almond butter
3–5 medjool dates, pitted
2 tbsp shelled hemp seeds
1 tsp ground cinnamon
½ tsp ground cloves

In a high-speed blender or food processor, combine all the ingredients and blend on high for 60–90 seconds, or until smooth and creamy.

Pour the smoothie into a glass and enjoy cold.

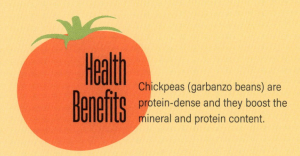

Health Benefits

Chickpeas (garbanzo beans) are protein-dense and they boost the mineral and protein content.

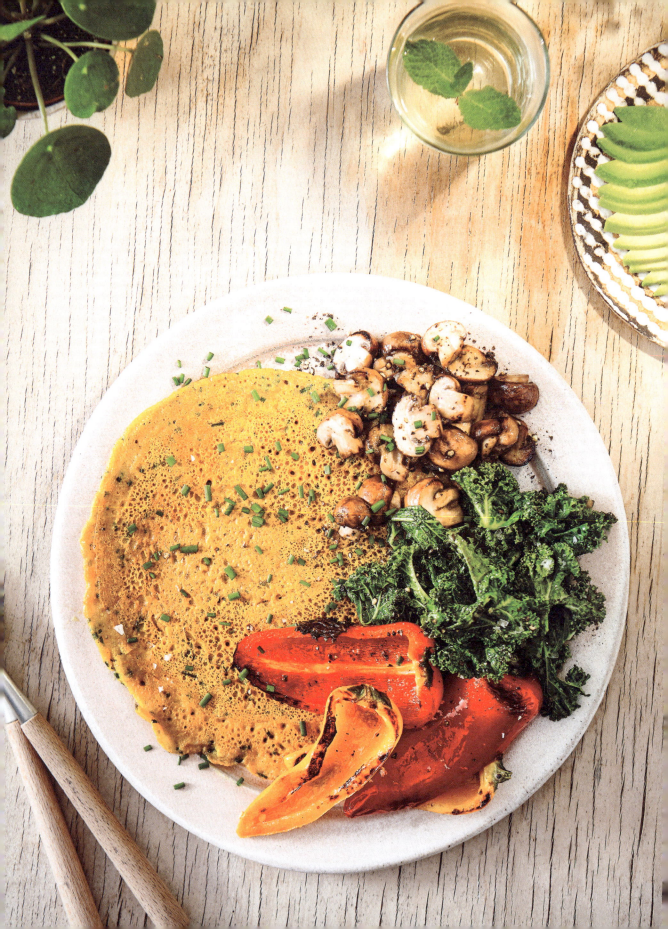

Chickpea Omelette

The first time I made this dish I was amazed at how effortless it is to enjoy a nutritious meal. The omelette takes less than 10 minutes to prepare and, when topped with hummus, avocado and spinach, it transforms into a complete, nourishing meal. Whether for breakfast, a quick lunch, or a wholesome dinner, this recipe adapts to your day effortlessly. It's one of my go-to meals, especially when I'm short on time. Plus, chickpea flour is packed with protein and fibre-rich carbs, making it perfect for those aiming to maintain weight or build muscle.

In a mixing bowl, combine the chickpea flour, salt, onion powder, garlic granules and turmeric. Mix well. Gradually add 80ml (2½fl oz/⅓ cup) water, while whisking continuously, until the batter is smooth and free of lumps.

Place a stainless-steel skillet or frying pan over a medium-high heat. Once hot, add the olive oil, ensuring the surface is evenly coated, and heat until it shimmers.

Pour in the batter, tilting the pan in circular motions to spread the batter evenly. Let the omelette cook undisturbed for 3–4 minutes. The batter may appear too wet, but it will firm up as it cooks.

Once the edges are dry and the centre is firm, carefully use a spatula to flip the omelette. Cook for an additional 1–2 minutes, until fully set and golden.

Spinkle with the chives and enjoy immediately, alongside avocado, leafy greens, mushrooms and peppers for a complete meal.

30g (1oz/⅓ cup) chickpea flour
1 tsp sea salt
1 tsp onion powder
1 tsp garlic granules
1 tsp ground turmeric
2 tbsp extra-virgin olive oil
Handful of fresh chives, finely diced (optional)

For Serving
Sliced avocado
Steamed leafy greens
Cooked mushrooms
Roasted peppers

Note
The batter should be slightly thicker than pancake batter. Adjust the water, if needed.

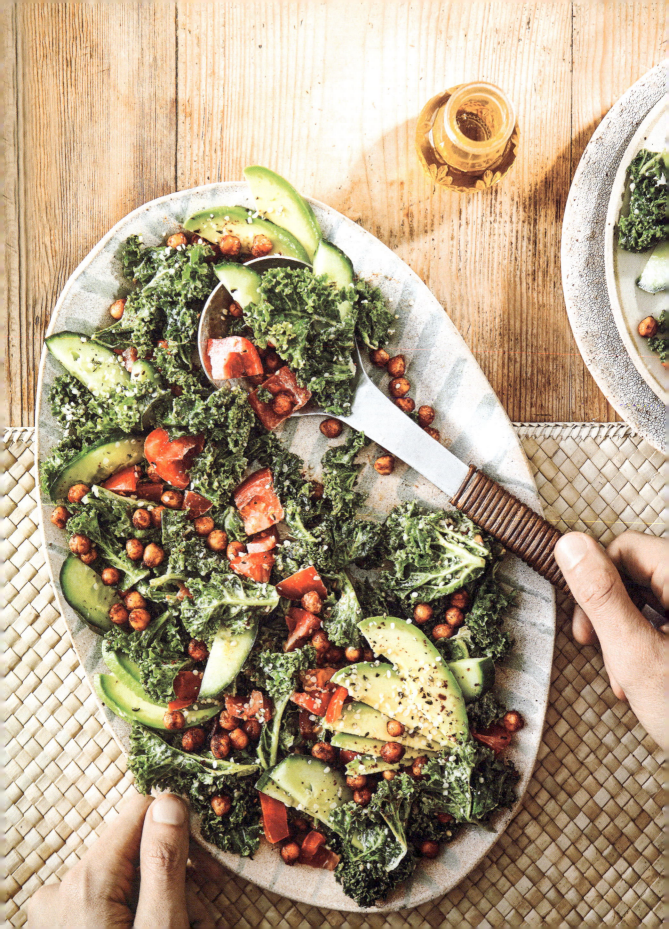

My Sister's Everyday Glow Salad

Serves 1–2
Prep 15 minutes
Cook 25 minutes

'Kids that grow kale, eat kale.' That's what Ron Finley said, and it stuck with me. But I'd add something – kids that know how to prepare kale, actually enjoy eating it. No one likes bland, undercooked chicken, right? That's why we season, marinate and cook it correctly. But when it comes to greens, people just toss them raw on a plate and wonder why they taste like punishment. Kale needs a little love. I learned this from my sister. She made this salad for lunch every single day and, eventually, she taught me the trick – massage the kale properly, let the seasonings do their work and, suddenly, kale isn't tough or bitter anymore, it's vibrant, fresh and full of flavour. Massaging breaks down the toughness, making it softer, easier to digest and better at absorbing nutrients. Add crispy, roasted chickpeas, creamy avocado and a drizzle of tahini, and you've got a simple, nourishing meal that actually hits. This will be your new go-to lunch – simple, satisfying and packed with everything your body needs.

Preheat the oven to Fan 180°C/200°C/400°F/Gas 6.

Spread the chickpeas on a clean towel and pat them dry. Place them in a bowl with the smoked paprika, cumin, cinnamon, maple syrup, salt, pepper and olive oil. Mix well to coat evenly.

Tip the chickpeas onto a baking tray and roast in the preheated oven for 20–25 minutes, shaking the tray halfway, until crispy and golden brown.

Meanwhile, place the chopped kale in a large bowl. Pour in the tahini, lime juice, maple syrup, olive oil and salt. Use your hands to massage the kale for about 4–5 minutes, working the dressing into the leaves until they just start to wilt.

Toss the cucumber, tomato and crispy chickpeas into the bowl with the kale, and mix well.

Divide the salad between two plates and top with the crispy chickpeas, sliced avocado and hemp or sesame seeds. Drizzle some extra tahini on top, if you like.

Crispy Chickpeas

1 x 400g (14oz) can chickpeas (garbanzo beans), drained and rinsed
1 tsp smoked paprika
1 tsp ground cumin
½ tsp ground cinnamon
1 tsp maple syrup
½ tsp sea salt
½ tsp black pepper
1 tbsp extra-virgin olive oil

Kale Salad

120g (4¼oz) kale, stalks removed and leaves chopped
2–3 tbsp tahini, plus extra for drizzling (optional)
Juice of 1 lime
1 tbsp maple syrup
2 tbsp extra-virgin olive oil
1 tsp sea salt
½ cucumber, chopped
1 Roma tomato, diced
1 avocado, sliced
1 tbsp shelled hemp seeds (or sesame seeds)

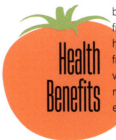

Health Benefits

Kale is packed with iron, fibre and antioxidants, and chickpeas (garbanzo beans) add protein and slow-digesting fibre, keeping you full and fuelled for hours. The combination of healthy fats from the tahini and avocado, and the vitamin C from the fresh lime juice, maintains your immune system and enhances iron absorption.

15-Minute Power Beans

Beans on toast – but not how you know them. This comes together in under 15 minutes, making it the perfect go-to for a quick brunch or satisfying lunch that actually fuels you. Butter beans are packed with protein, fibre and slow-releasing energy, keeping you full and steady for hours. Simmered with garlic, warming spices and a hit of lime, they turn creamy and full of flavour. A swirl of tahini brings it all together, adding richness and depth. Simple, nourishing and seriously good.

Pour a generous drizzle of olive oil into a pan over a medium heat. Add the garlic, smoked paprika, cayenne, cumin and tomato purée. Sauté for 2–3 minutes until fragrant.

Add the butter beans and a splash of water, and cook for 5–7 minutes, stirring occasionally, until heated through and bubbling.

Remove from the heat, stir in the tahini and squeeze in the lime juice. Season with salt and pepper to taste.

Spoon the creamy butter beans on top of the sourdough toast and finish with your favourite toppings, such as chilli flakes, avocado or fresh herbs.

Drizzle of extra-virgin olive oil
2 garlic cloves, finely chopped
1 tsp smoked paprika
½ tsp cayenne pepper (adjust to taste)
½ tsp ground cumin
1 tbsp tomato purée (paste)
1 x 400g (14oz) can butter (lima) beans, drained and rinsed
1 tbsp tahini
Juice of 1 lime
Sea salt and black pepper

For Serving

2 slices sourdough bread, toasted
Chilli (red pepper) flakes (optional)
Avocado (optional)
Fresh herbs of your choice (optional)

Health Benefits

Butter (lima) beans are a powerhouse of plant-based protein, fibre and slow-digesting carbs – keeping you full, energised and balanced. The garlic and spices contain natural antioxidants while the lime juice adds vitamin C to further support the healthy functioning of our immune system.

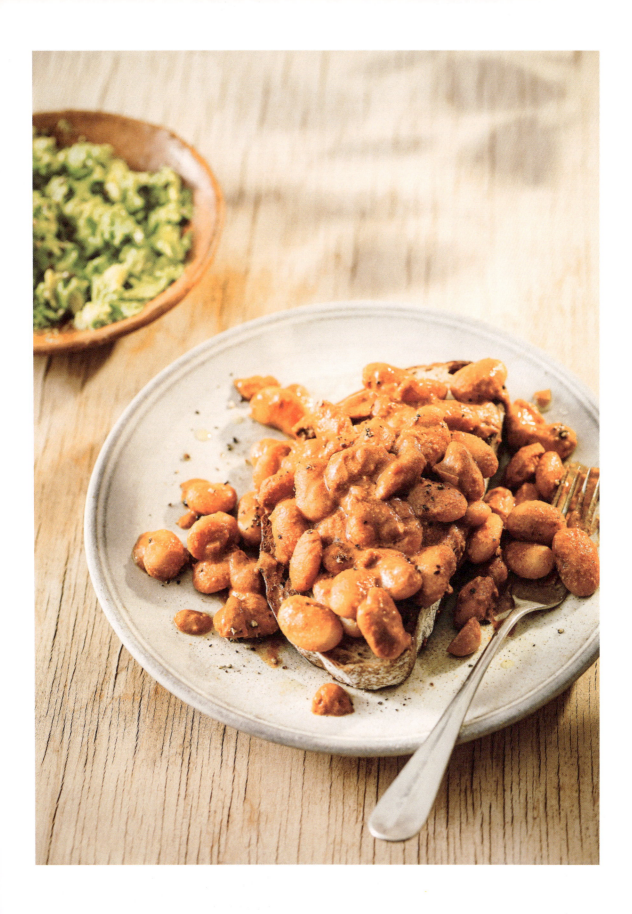

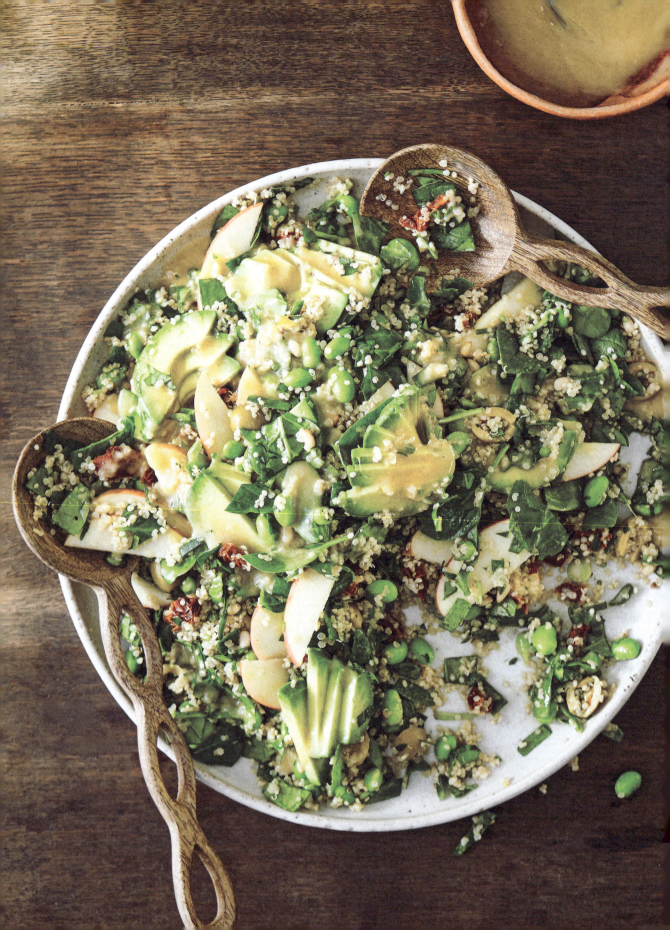

To-Go 20 Minute Power Bowl

Serves 1–2
Prep 15 minutes
Cook 20 minutes

Lunch break. Twenty minutes. No clue what to cook? This is your answer. A power-packed bowl that fuels you through the day, keeping you full, energised and feeling good. With quinoa as the protein base, crunchy pine nuts, briny olives and sun-dried tomatoes for depth, this salad is anything but boring. Topped with creamy avocado and tossed in a vibrant lemon-tahini dressing with a touch of sweetness, this is the kind of meal that makes healthy eating effortless, even when you're on the go.

Place the quinoa in a pot with 475ml (17fl oz/2 cups) water. Bring to a boil, then reduce the heat and simmer gently for about 15 minutes, or until all the water is absorbed.

Remove from heat, cover and set aside for 5 minutes before fluffing with a fork.

Meanwhile, place a dry frying pan over a medium heat. Add the pine nuts and toast for about 2–3 minutes, stirring frequently, until golden and fragrant. Be careful – they burn easily. Transfer to a plate to cool.

In a small bowl, make the dressing by whisking together all the ingredients. Adjust the seasoning to taste.

In a large bowl, combine the quinoa, edamame, spinach, parsley, spring onions, olives, sun-dried tomatoes, finely chopped apple and toasted pine nuts. Drizzle the dressing over the top and toss until everything is well coated.

Divide into bowls, top with the avocado slices and enjoy immediately, or refrigerate for later.

185g (6½oz) quinoa, rinsed

30g (1oz) pine nuts

250g (9oz) cooked edamame or cannellini beans

150g (5½oz) baby spinach, roughly chopped

15g (½oz) flat-leaf parsley, chopped

3 spring onions (scallions), chopped

50g (1¾oz) pitted green olives, halved

50g (1¾oz) sun-dried tomatoes, chopped

1 apple, cored and finely chopped

1 ripe avocado, thinly sliced

Lemon-Tahini Dressing

4 tbsp olive oil

3 tbsp fresh lemon juice (adjust to taste)

2 tbsp tahini

1 tbsp maple syrup

1 large garlic clove, minced

½ tsp sea salt

Black pepper

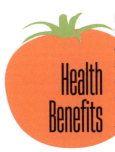

Health Benefits

This bowl is a powerhouse of nutrients. Quinoa delivers complete plant-based protein, containing all nine essential amino acids, making it a great part of a balanced meal. Edamame is another complete protein and is also fibre rich, while olives and sun-dried tomatoes provide healthy plant chemicals, as well as a rich, satisfying, umami flavour. Pine nuts bring a dose of healthy fats and fibre, as does avocado, helping to keep you feeling full for longer. The addition of apple adds a refreshing crunch and natural sweetness. This salad is perfect for meal prep – it keeps well in the fridge for up to 3 days, and the flavours get even better over time. Don't add the avocado until ready to eat to prevent browning.

Chuna

I'm not usually a fan of modern alternatives to classic foods, but this recipe is simply irresistible. I combined the creamy texture of chickpeas with the citrusy zest of dill and lemon juice, the pungency of onions, the sweetness of maple syrup, and the saltiness of nori flakes. The result is a burst of flavour that will have you coming back for more. Serve it on romaine lettuce or sourdough bread for the perfect lunch, side dish or snack.

Add the chickpeas to a large mixing bowl. Using a potato masher or fork, mash the chickpeas for 2–3 minutes, until they reach your desired texture. You can leave some chunks for a heartier consistency or mash them completely for a smoother base.

Add all the remaining ingredients to the bowl and mix thoroughly until everything is well combined.

Serve the chuna on lettuce leaves or sourdough toast with pickled red onions and guacamole, if desired.

300g (10½oz) cooked chickpeas (garbanzo beans)
½ red onion, finely diced
5 tbsp tahini
1 tbsp fresh lemon juice
1 tbsp dried dill
1 tsp onion powder
1 tsp maple syrup
1 tsp sea salt
3 tbsp nori flakes
2 tbsp tamari (or coconut aminos)

For Serving (optional)
Romaine lettuce
2–4 slices sourdough bread, toasted
Pickled red onions
Guacamole (see page 99)

Note
This versatile mixture can also be used as a sandwich or wrap filling.

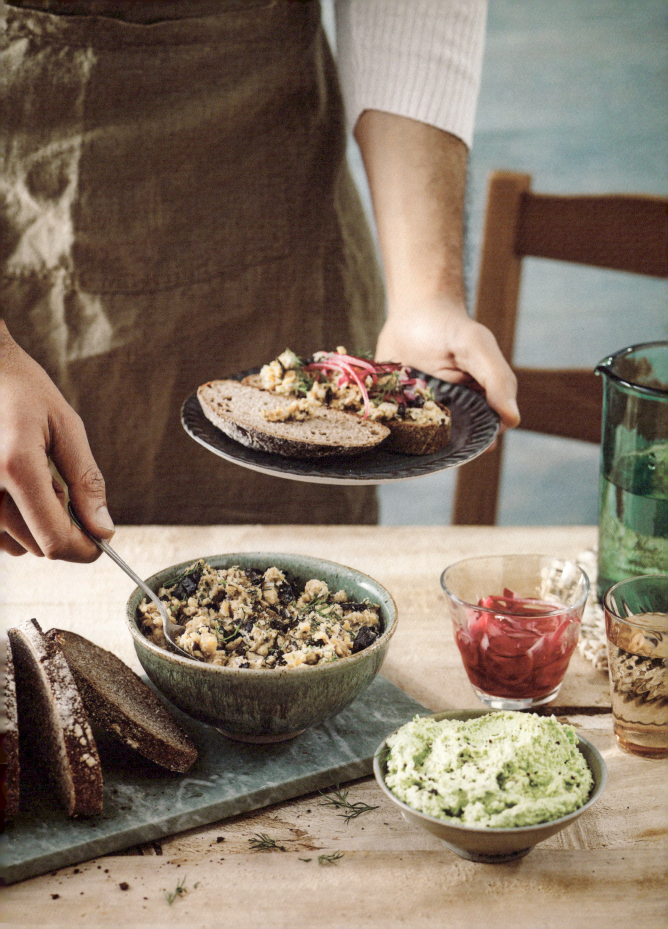

Edamame Power Smash

Who said plant-based meals can't be protein powerhouses? This edamame smash delivers approximately 30g (1oz) protein per serving when loaded onto sourdough bread with hemp seeds. It's creamy, savoury and packed with nutrients that fuel your body without any fuss. Edamame is one of the best plant-based protein sources, delivering all nine essential amino acids. Tahini and hemp seeds add extra healthy fats, minerals and plant protein, while the lime and coriander bring fresh, detoxifying benefits. Perfect for post-workout recovery or just a solid, energy-packed meal.

In a high-speed blender or food processor, combine the edamame, tahini, avocado, maple syrup, garlic, cayenne pepper, coriander, sesame oil, lime juice and salt. Blend until it forms a thick paste.

Spread on the toasted sourdough and sprinkle with the hemp seeds. Add some sauerkraut or pickled onions for extra nutrients.

350g (12oz) shelled frozen edamame, defrosted
60g (2¼oz) tahini
½ ripe avocado
1 tsp maple syrup
4 garlic cloves, roughly chopped
½ tsp cayenne pepper (or to taste)
Handful of fresh coriander (cilantro)
1 tsp toasted sesame oil
Juice of 1 lime
1 tsp sea salt
1–2 slices sourdough bread, toasted
2–3 tbsp shelled hemp seeds
Sauerkraut or pickled onions, to serve (optional)

Note
Keep any leftovers in an airtight container in the fridge for up to 7 days.

The Best Hummus

Serves 4–5
Prep 10 minutes
Cook 2 minutes

Once you've made hummus from scratch, there's no going back. Store-bought just doesn't compare – too thick, too pasty, or missing that fresh, rich flavour that only comes from real ingredients. On my visit to Egypt, I had the best hummus of my life – so smooth it changed my expectations of hummus forever. A Syrian chef explained the process to me step-by-step, breaking down exactly what makes the difference – nutty tahini, bright lemon, slow-cooked garlic-infused olive oil, all blended into a dip so creamy it practically melts on your tongue. One scoop, then another and, before you know it, the bowl is empty.

Place the chickpeas in a food processor and blend for 1–2 minutes until smooth and thick. Scrape down the sides, as needed, to ensure everything is evenly processed.

Add the tahini, fresh lemon juice, chopped garlic, cumin, and salt and pepper to taste. Blend again until well combined.

With the motor running, slowly drizzle in 6–8 tablespoons ice-cold water, a tablespoon at a time, until the hummus becomes light, creamy and velvety. The ice water helps achieve a smooth texture. Scrape down the sides, taste and adjust seasoning as needed. Blend one last time for extra smoothness.

To make the topping, if using, heat the extra-virgin olive oil in a small pan over a low heat. Once warm, add the thinly sliced garlic and lemon peel. Sizzle gently for about 2 minutes until golden – be careful not to let them burn. Sprinkle in a little salt, then remove the garlic and lemon zest from the oil.

Pour the warm, infused oil over the hummus, then top with the crispy garlic and lemon peel, a pinch of paprika and some freshly chopped parsley.

Serve the hummus with homemade naan, flatbread, or crunchy veggies.

225g (8oz) cooked chickpeas (garbanzo beans)
190g (6½oz) tahini
5–7 tbsp fresh lemon juice
3 garlic cloves, chopped
1 tsp ground cumin
6–8 tbsp ice-cold water
Sea salt and black pepper

Toppings (optional)
4–5 tbsp extra-virgin olive oil
3–4 garlic cloves, sliced into long, thin slivers
5 thin strips of organic lemon peel
Pinch of paprika
Small bunch of parsley, chopped

For Serving (optional)
Naan or flatbread
Crunchy vegetables

Notes
The key to next-level hummus is quality ingredients. Use 100 per cent sesame tahini (no added oils) and a high-quality extra-virgin olive oil for the best flavour. For the dreamiest texture, peeling the chickpea skins makes a difference – but it's optional. Cooking dried chickpeas from scratch gives the creamiest result, but canned works, too – just rinse them well.

SHINE

79

Creamy Mushroom & Chickpea Pasta

Serves 3–4
Prep 10 minutes
Cook 20 minutes

Mushrooms are more like us than we think. Unlike plants, they don't photosynthesise – instead, they breathe oxygen and convert organic material into energy, just like we do. Some theories even suggest that mushrooms are nature's original internet, communicating through vast underground networks that connect entire ecosystems. When it comes to food, they're just as fascinating. Loaded with immune-boosting beta-glucans, essential minerals like selenium and zinc, and compounds that support brain function, mushrooms are a nutritional powerhouse. In this dish, they bring their signature umami depth, turning a simple pasta into something rich, hearty, and deeply nourishing.

To make the sauce, place all the ingredients in a high-speed blender or food processor and blend until smooth. Adjust the consistency by adding more milk, if needed, to achieve a smooth and pourable sauce. Set aside.

Put the olive oil in a large pan over a medium heat. Add the onion, garlic, spring onions and thyme with a pinch of salt. Cook for 5–7 minutes until soft and translucent, stirring occasionally to avoid burning.

Meanwhile, bring a pot of salted water to a boil and cook the pasta according to the packet instructions. Drain and set aside.

Once the onion mixutre is fragrant, add the sliced mushrooms and chickpeas to the pan and cook for 5 minutes, until the mushrooms soften and release their juices. Stir in the spinach and fresh basil, letting them wilt into the mixture.

Pour the creamy sauce into the pan with the vegetables and stir well, letting it warm through for 2–3 minutes. Add the drained pasta, tossing everything together until it's well coated.

Adjust the seasoning to taste, then serve immediately, topped with some fresh basil or a sprinkle of toasted pine nuts, if using.

2 tsp extra-virgin olive oil
1 small brown onion, finely chopped
4 garlic cloves, minced
2 spring onions (scallions), finely chopped
1 tsp dried thyme
Pinch of sea salt
250g (9oz) pasta of choice (spelt, lentil or buckwheat work well)
250g (9oz) mushrooms (button, oyster, portobello, or shiitake), sliced
1 × 400g (14oz) can chickpeas (garbanzo beans), drained and rinsed
2 handfuls of spinach
1 handful of fresh basil, chopped, plus extra to garnish
1 tbsp pine nuts, toasted (optional)

Creamy Nut Sauce

200g (7oz) Brazil nuts or cashews (or shelled hemp seeds for a nut-free option), soaked for 2–4 hours, then drained (see page 25)
1 tbsp onion powder
1 tsp garlic powder
250–300ml (9–10fl oz/generous 1 cup) unsweetened milk of choice (coconut or almond work well)
1 tsp maple syrup
Juice of ½ lemon
1 tbsp almond butter
1 tsp sea salt
Black pepper
Pinch of cayenne pepper (optional)

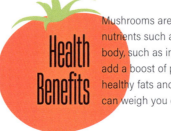

Health Benefits

Mushrooms are a brilliant nutrient dense-food – low in energy but high in nutrients such as vitamins and fibre. These nutrients support systems within our body, such as immunity, gut health and brain health. Chickpeas (garbanzo beans) add a boost of plant-based protein and fibre, while the creamy sauce provides healthy fats and minerals to keep you fuelled. Unlike traditional creamy pasta that can weigh you down, this dish is light and easy to digest, but sustaining.

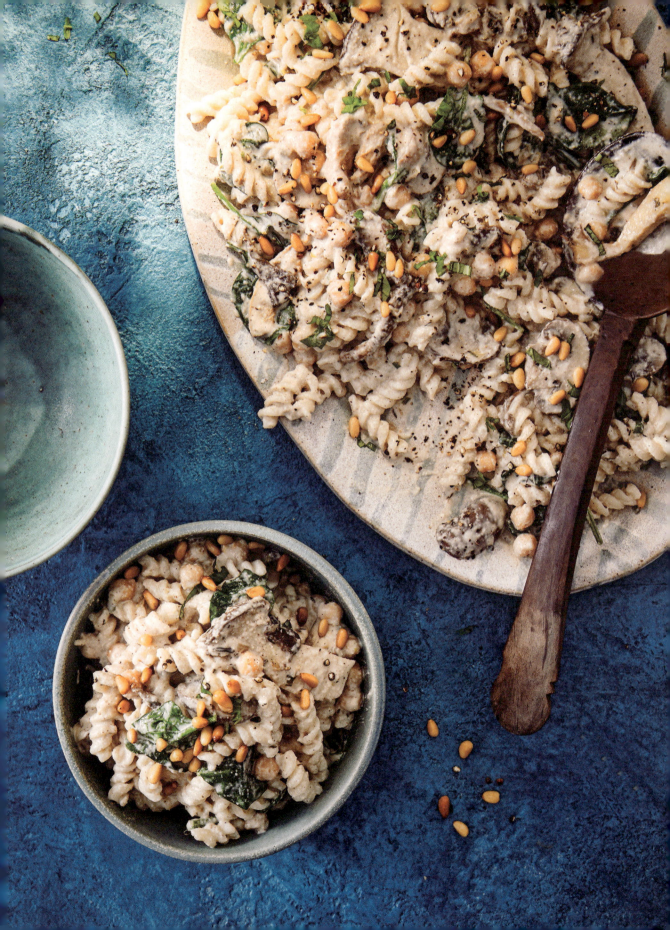

One-Pot Quinoa Chickpea Meal

Serves 2
Prep 5 minutes
Cook 50 minutes

This is one of my meal-prep favourites. And the best part? Everything can be prepared in one pot. Simple, yet effective – that's what I'm all about when it comes to busy weekdays. I want something nourishing, without breaking the bank or spending hours cooking and cleaning countless dishes. I love prepping this and storing it in containers in the fridge, so when I get home tired, I have a healthy, wholesome dinner waiting for me.

To make the spiced chickpeas, heat the extra-virgin olive oil in a large skillet or frying pan over a medium heat. Add the chickpeas and fry for 4–5 minutes, stirring occasionally, until golden and crispy. Sprinkle with cayenne pepper, onion powder, smoked paprika and salt, and cook for another 3–4 minutes, allowing the chickpeas to absorb the spices. Transfer to a plate and set aside.

Using the same skillet or pan, make the quinoa base. Add the extra-virgin olive oil, chopped onion and salt, and cook over a medium heat for 4–5 minutes until the onion softens and caramelises.

Reduce the heat to medium-low, stir in the chopped ginger, and fry for 2–3 minutes.

Add the passata, stirring well, and cook for 2 minutes.

Add the rinsed quinoa, along with the basil, oregano, onion powder and allspice. Stir well to coat the quinoa in all the flavours. Pour in 360ml (12fl oz/1½ cups) water and increase the heat to bring to a boil. Reduce the heat, cover with a lid and simmer for 20–25 minutes, or until the quinoa has absorbed the liquid.

Fold in the crispy chickpeas and all the toppings. Mix well to combine and serve warm.

Spiced Chickpeas

1 tbsp extra-virgin olive oil
240g (8½oz) cooked chickpeas
(garbanzo beans)
1 tsp cayenne pepper
1 tsp onion powder
½ tsp smoked paprika
½ tsp sea salt

Quinoa Base

2 tbsp extra-virgin olive oil
80g (2¾oz) brown onion, chopped
½ tsp sea salt
1 tbsp finely grated fresh root ginger
180ml (6fl oz) passata
170g (6oz) quinoa, rinsed
1 tsp dried basil
1 tsp dried oregano
1 tsp onion powder
½ tsp ground allspice

Toppings

15g (½oz) fresh coriander (cilantro),
chopped
50g (1¾oz) sun-dried tomatoes,
chopped
30g (1oz) raisins or dates, finely
chopped

Quick Green Pesto

If you're after a quick weekday recipe packed with veggies, this one's for you. In just 15 minutes, you'll have a nourishing meal that tastes incredible. The best part? You can get creative with the ingredients. No cashews? Swap them for pine nuts or walnuts. No basil? Try spinach or kale instead. This recipe proves that veggies can work with you, not against you!

In a high-speed blender or food processor, combine all the ingredients. Add 4 tablespoons water and blend until smooth and creamy. Season with salt and pepper to taste, blending briefly to incorporate.

Serve the pesto with spelt or gluten-free pasta.

75g (2¾oz) cashews

1 ripe avocado

Zest and juice of 1 lemon

1 large handful basil leaves (about 30g/1oz)

5 tbsp extra-virgin olive oil

2 sun-dried tomatoes

2 garlic cloves

Sea salt and black pepper

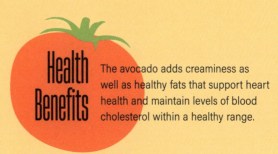

Health Benefits The avocado adds creaminess as well as healthy fats that support heart health and maintain levels of blood cholesterol within a healthy range.

Glow-Up Pesto

The best things in life are simple. Pesto is proof that a handful of fresh ingredients can create something powerful. This isn't just a sauce – it's a blend of deep greens, brain-fuelling walnuts and vibrant flavours that would bring any dish to life. The kale and spinach pack in the nutrients, while the walnuts give it a rich, earthy backbone. A quick blitz and you've got a bold, nourishing and incredibly versatile staple that belongs on everything – grains, roasted veg, pasta, or toast. Once you start making this at home, there's no turning back.

In a high-speed blender or food processor, combine all the ingredients and pulse for 15–20 seconds until everything is evenly chopped and combined. If you prefer a chunky pesto, keep it as is. For a smoother consistency, blend for longer, adding a splash more olive oil, if needed.

Taste to check the seasoning – add more salt, a little extra olive oil, or even another handful of basil, if you want it more fragrant.

100g (3½oz) spinach
90g (3¼oz) kale, stalks removed
40g (1½oz) fresh basil
200g (7oz) walnuts
100g (3½oz) cooked edamame
6–7 tbsp extra-virgin olive oil
1 tsp sea salt (adjust to taste)

Note
If you're not using the pesto immediately, spoon it into a glass jar and top it with a light drizzle of olive oil to keep it fresh. Seal it and store in the fridge for up to 4 days. You can also freeze it for up to 3 months.

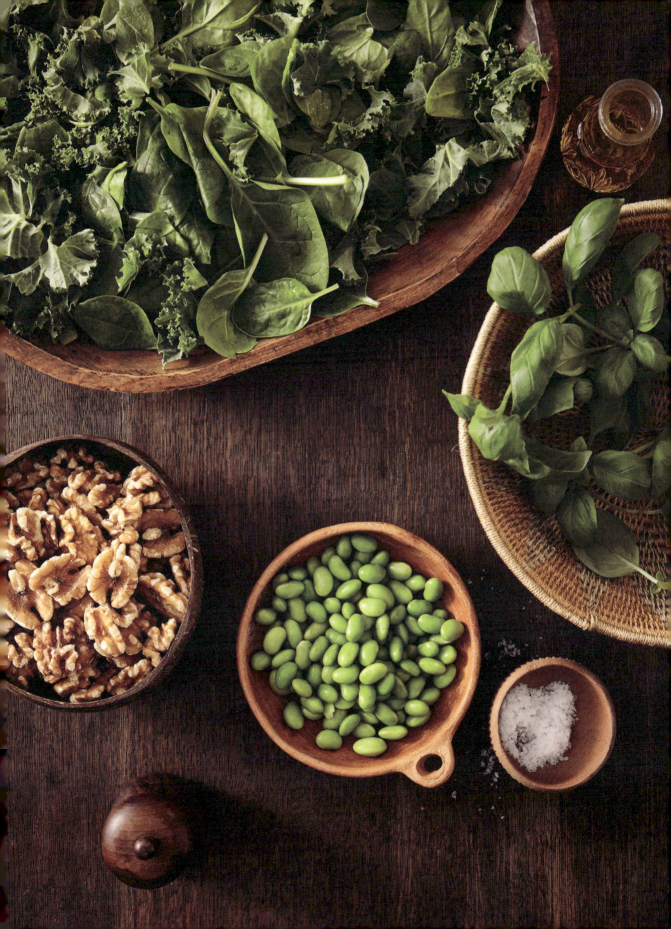

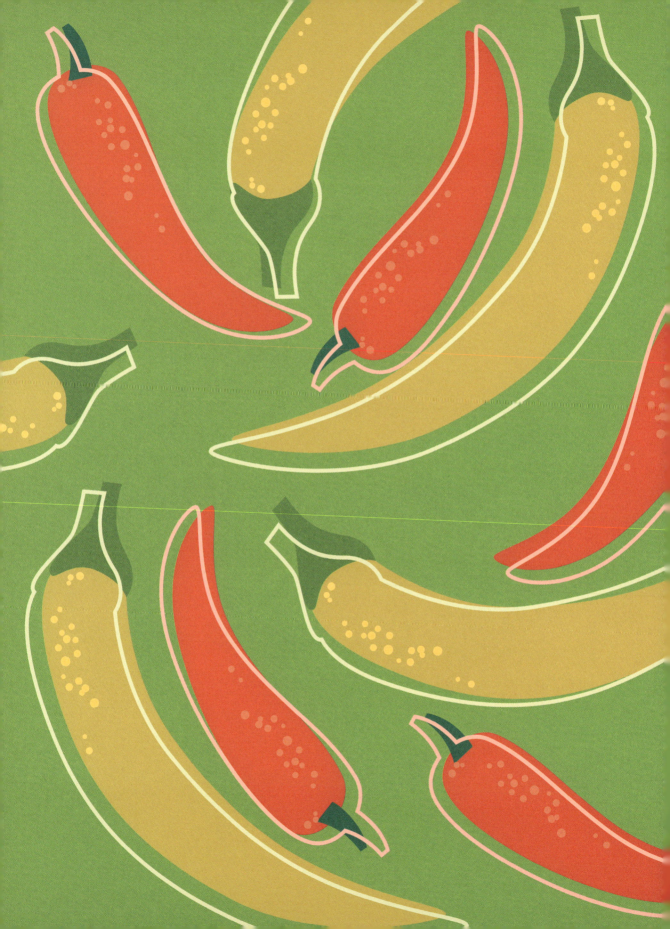

REPLENISHING DINNERS

RESTORE

Smoky Chipotle–Spiced Tofu

Serves 3–4
Prep 12 minutes
Cook 1 hour 5 minutes

I've always believed that tofu is only as good as what you do with it. Leave it bland, and it's forgettable – but treat it right, and it soaks up every bit of flavour. This is the kind of dish you make for friends. Bold, smoky and packed with deep flavour, this has that slow-cooked taste with minimal effort. Serve it burrito bowl-style with coriander rice or quinoa, guacamole and black beans, and you've got a meal that hits every spot.

To roast the green bell pepper using a gas stove or grill (broiler), place the pepper directly over an open flame or under the grill, turning every 30–60 seconds with tongs until the skin is charred all over. This should take around 4–5 minutes. Set aside to cool slightly before removing the stem and seeds.

To roast the pepper using the oven method, preheat the oven to Fan 200°C/220°C/425°F/Gas 7. Rub the pepper with 1 teaspoon of the oil and place it on a baking tray. Roast for 20–25 minutes, turning halfway through, until softened and slightly charred. Let it cool slightly before removing the stem and seeds.

In a frying pan, heat 2 tablespoons of the oil over a medium-high heat. Add the chopped onion and a small pinch of salt and cook for 5–6 minutes, stirring occasionally, until it turns soft and golden. Stir in the garlic and cook for 2 minutes, stirring frequently so it doesn't burn.

Add the tomato purée, cumin, oregano, cayenne pepper, and salt and black pepper and let everything cook for about 1 minute to bring out the flavours.

Add the chopped tomatoes and cook for 5 minutes, stirring occasionally, until they soften. Remove the pan from the from heat.

Meanwhile, drain the tofu, pat it dry and squeeze out any moisture. Crumble it with your hands into small, uneven chunks about the size of a raisin.

Transfer the cooked onion and tomato mixture to a high-speed blender or food processor. Add the roasted bell pepper, the sun-dried tomatoes, date or maple syrup and just enough water to make a smooth texture (about 3½ tablespoons). Blend well, then taste and adjust the seasoning, if needed.

Return the frying pan to the heat, add the remaining oil and, once hot, spread out the crumbled tofu in an even layer. Sprinkle with 1 teaspoon salt and let it cook, without stirring, for 2–3 minutes. Stir, then continue cooking for 7–8 minutes, stirring every few minutes, until golden and slightly crispy.

Pour the blended sauce over the tofu and stir to coat. Simmer over a medium heat for 5 minutes, then lower the heat and cook for another 5–6 minutes, stirring occasionally. Finish with a squeeze of fresh lime juice and fresh coriander and serve with sliced avocado, diced mango and pickled red onions.

1 green bell pepper
4 tbsp avocado oil or extra-virgin olive oil
1 red onion, finely chopped
4 garlic cloves, chopped
2 tbsp tomato purée (paste)
1½ tsp ground cumin
1 tsp dried oregano
½ tsp cayenne pepper
2 medium-large tomatoes, chopped
400–450g (14oz–1lb) firm tofu
4–5 sun-dried tomatoes in oil, drained
2 tbsp date syrup (or 2 tsp maple syrup)
Juice of 1 lime
Handful of fresh coriander (cilantro), chopped
Sea salt and black pepper

For Serving
Sliced avocado
Diced mango
Picked red onions

Notes
Super firm tofu works best here, as it holds its texture, but if you're using extra firm, just press out any excess water first. This dish is a meal-prep dream – it tastes even better the next day.

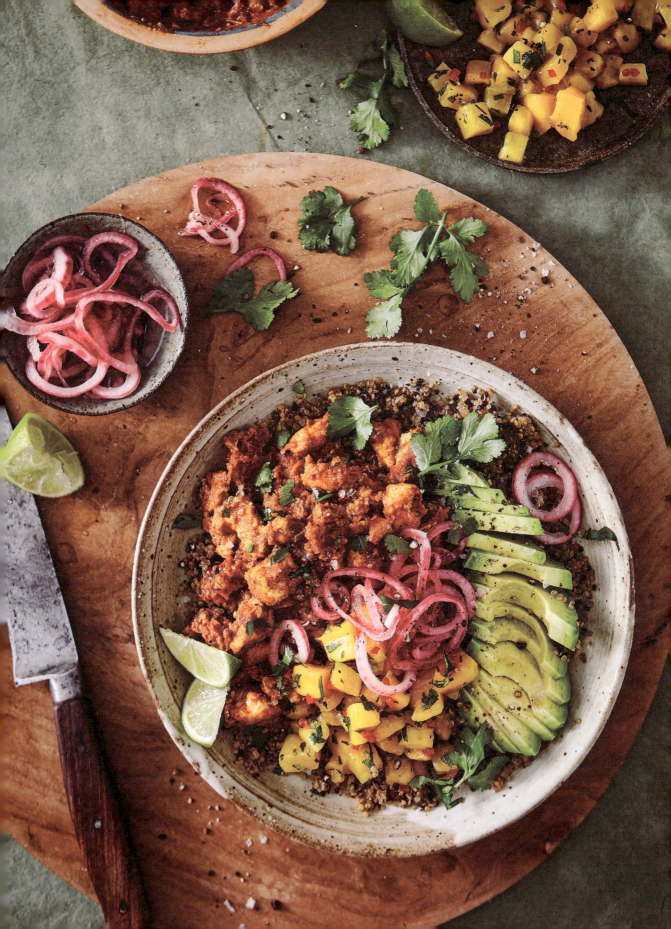

Broccoli & Butter Bean Power Stir

Serves 2
Prep 5 minutes
Cook 15 minutes

This dish is one I turn to when life gets hectic, but I still want to feel grounded and nourished. I remember throwing it together after a long day, using whatever I had in the kitchen – broccoli, a can of chickpeas and some cashews for crunch. The result was so satisfying that it quickly became a weeknight staple. It's proof that wholesome meals don't have to be complicated. With just a few ingredients and one pan, you've got a vibrant, nutrient-packed dinner that makes you feel as good as it tastes.

In a small bowl, mix together the vegetable stock, sesame oil, tamari and flour, if using. If you enjoy heat, stir in some cayenne to taste.

Place a large skillet or frying pan over a medium heat and add the olive oil. Toss in the minced garlic and sauté for about 1 minute, until fragrant – don't let it burn.

Add the broccoli and pour in the sauce. Stir until the broccoli is well coated, then lower the heat to medium-low, cover with a lid and cook for about 6–8 minutes, stirring every so often to prevent sticking. If it starts to dry out, add a splash of vegetable stock.

Once the broccoli is nearly cooked, stir in the cashews and butter beans or chickpeas. Cover the pan again and cook for another 4–6 minutes.

Remove from the heat and serve immediately over your base of choice – I love serving this with steamed quinoa or rice.

4 tbsp vegetable stock

2 tbsp toasted sesame oil

5 tbsp tamari (or coconut aminos)

1 tbsp spelt, chickpea, or almond flour (optional, to thicken sauce)

½–1 tsp cayenne pepper (optional)

3 tbsp extra-virgin olive oil

6–8 garlic cloves, minced

1 head of broccoli, broken into florets

115g (4oz) cashews, chopped

250g (9oz) cooked butter (lima) beans or chickpeas (garbanzo beans)

For Serving

Steamed quinoa or rice

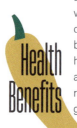

Health Benefits

Broccoli, the star of this dish, is a powerhouse of antioxidants and vitamin C, vitamin K and folic acid. Some of the nutrients support the healthy functioning of our immune system, and may help reduce chronic inflammation. Butter (lima) beans and chickpeas (garbanzo beans) bring plant-based protein and fibre, helping to keep you full and your digestion running smoothly. Cashews not only add crunch but also provide healthy fats, magnesium, zinc and fibre for sustained release of energy. This is more than just a stir-fry, it's a nutrient-packed bowl of goodness to keep you feeling vibrant and strong.

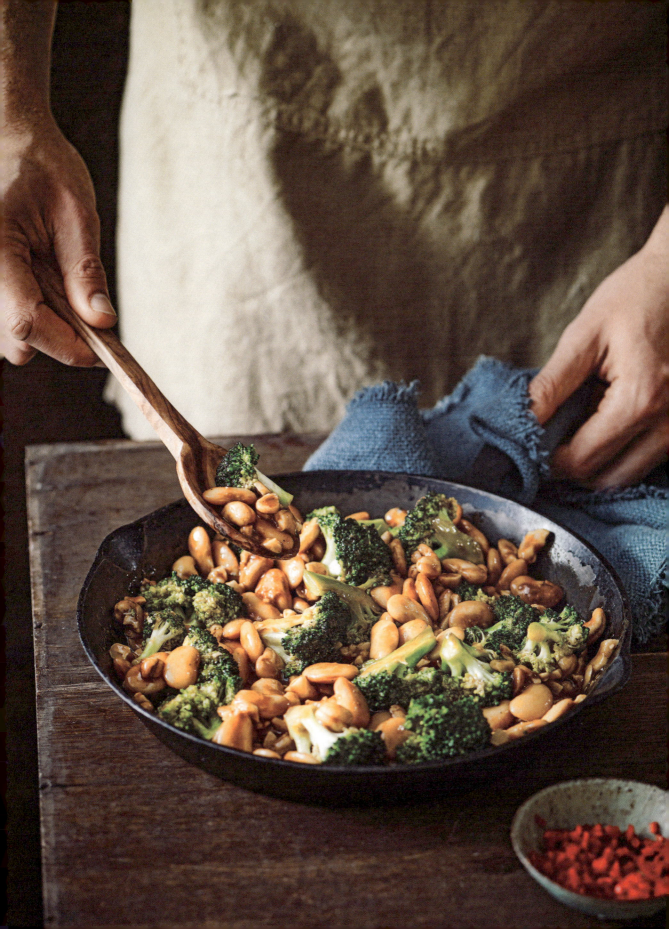

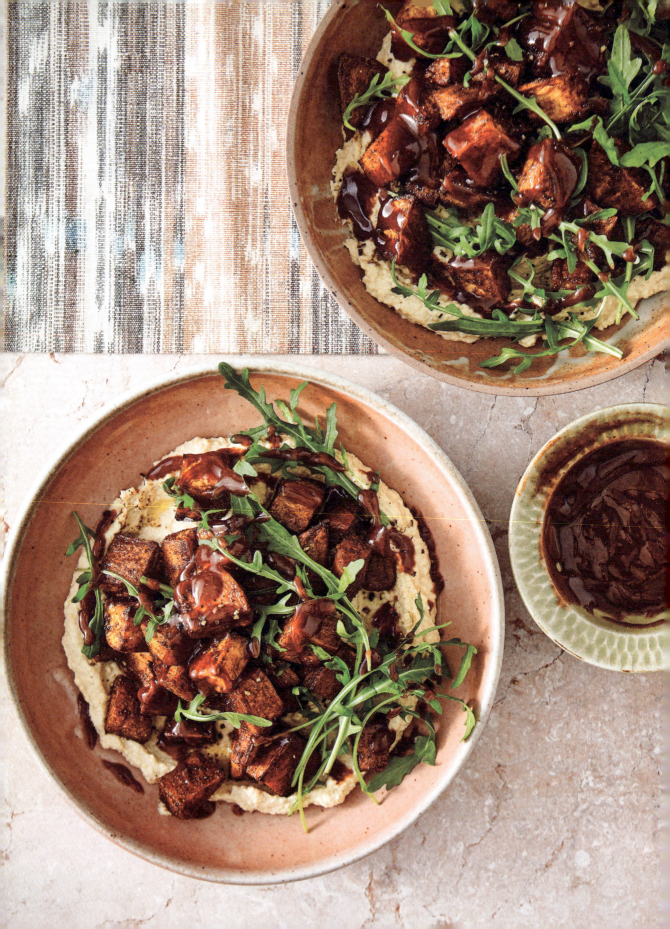

The Earth Bowl

Every bite we take is either building us up or slowing us down. This bowl does the former – loaded with fibre, healthy fats and plant-based protein, it fuels your body with everything it needs to thrive. Sweet potatoes bring natural sweetness and slow-burning energy, while almond butter and sesame oil create a creamy, spiced glaze that takes them to another level. Paired with hummus for extra protein and rocket for a peppery bite, this dish is a powerhouse of nutrients wrapped up in pure comfort. One bowl, endless benefits.

Preheat the oven to Fan 180°C/200°C/400°F/Gas 6.

Spread the sweet potato chunks on a baking tray, drizzle with the olive or avocado oil, then sprinkle over the cloves, cinnamon, cumin and salt. Season with some pepper and toss everything together until evenly coated. Roast in the preheated oven for 40–50 minutes, turning halfway, until soft and caramelised.

Meanwhile, in a bowl, whisk the dressing ingredients together with a pinch of salt until smooth and creamy. Add a tiny splash of water to loosen it, if needed.

Toss the roasted sweet potatoes in the dressing until well coated.

Spread a generous layer of hummus onto a serving plate, then pile the sweet potato on top. Scatter with the rocket and enjoy warm on its own or alongside some fresh flatbread or quinoa.

Spiced Sweet Potatoes

2 large sweet potatoes, peeled and cut into small chunks
2 tbsp extra-virgin olive or avocado oil
½ tsp ground cloves
1 tsp ground cinnamon
2 tsp ground cumin
1 tsp sea salt
Black pepper

Almond Sesame Dressing

2 tbsp date syrup (or 1 tbsp maple syrup)
3 tbsp toasted sesame oil
3 tbsp almond butter
Juice of ½ lemon

For Serving

A generous base of *The Best Hummus* (see page 79)
Handful of wild rocket (arugula)
Fresh flatbread or steamed quinoa (optional)

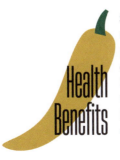

Health Benefits

Sweet potatoes are packed with beta-carotene, which has a really important role in maintaining healthy skin and a healthy immunue system. The hummus provides plant-based protein and fibre, keeping you full and slowly releasing energy, while the almond butter and sesame oil deliver healthy fats that help keep your heart healthy. The spices don't just add depth; when consumed regularly the naturally occuring chemicals within them may help reduce inflammation. Together, it's a complete, nourishing meal that fuels the body while tasting like pure comfort.

The Nourishment Bowl

'Man is what he eats,' as Ludwig Feuerbach once said. And who wouldn't want to embody the vibrancy of a nourishing bowl packed with natural goodness? A well-rounded salad brings together the essentials: colourful veggies, healthy fats, quality protein and plenty of fibre. This recipe delivers all that and more. One of my favourite things about it? The flavours deepen and come alive the next day. Just store it in the fridge and it's ready to serve as a satisfying main or side dish on those busy weeknights. Nourish to flourish.

To make the dressing, in a large mixing bowl, whisk together the lemon juice, garlic, salt, black pepper and cayenne pepper. Gradually drizzle in the olive oil, whisking all the time, until the mixture is smooth and well combined. Taste and adjust the seasoning. Set aside.

Place the lentils in a pot and cover with about 750ml (26fl oz/3¾ cups) water (enough to submerge them by at least 2–3cm/¾–1¼in). Add the bay leaves and bring to a gentle boil over a medium-high heat. Reduce the heat to low, cover with a lid and simmer for 20–25 minutes, or until the lentils are tender but still slightly firm. Drain thoroughly using a fine mesh strainer and discard the bay leaves.

While the lentils are still warm, transfer to the bowl with the dressing. Toss gently to ensure every lentil is coated with the vibrant flavours. Set aside to cool slightly.

Once the lentils have cooled (warm is fine, but not hot), add the cucumber, bell peppers, spring onions, parsley and mint. Toss everything gently to combine, making sure the dressing is evenly distributed.

Taste and adjust the seasoning or add more lemon juice to brighten it up, if desired. Serve immediately, or cover and store in the fridge for up to 3 days. This dish tastes even better after a couple of hours in the fridge.

200g (7oz/1 cup) black or green lentils, rinsed

2 bay leaves

1 cucumber, diced

1 red bell pepper, deseeded and finely chopped

1 orange bell pepper, deseeded and finely chopped

2 spring onions (scallions), finely chopped

20g (¾oz) fresh parsley, chopped

20g (¾oz) fresh mint, chopped

Dressing

5 tbsp fresh lemon juice (about 2 lemons)

3–4 garlic cloves, minced

1 tsp sea salt (adjust to taste)

½ tsp freshly ground black pepper (adjust to taste)

½ tsp cayenne pepper

5 tbsp extra-virgin olive oil

Health Benefits

In need of a little boost? Lentils are a great source of folic acid, which keeps blood vessels and arteries healthy, and selenium, which is good for brain and heart support.

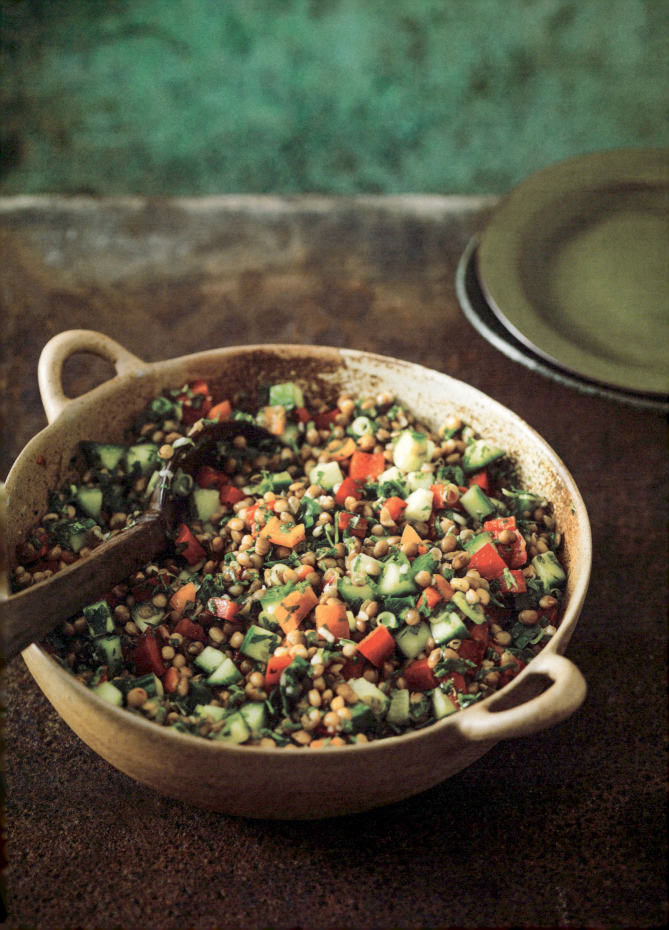

The Go-To Dal

If I could only cook one dish to convince a sceptic of the joys of unprocessed food, it would be this one. Thirty minutes, one pot and a handful of affordable pantry staples – that's all it takes to cook up a batch big enough to have your weeknight dinners sorted. Not many things in life give you this much comfort for so little effort. This dal is comfort in a bowl, simple and satisfying. Pair it with sweet potatoes or quinoa, some leafy greens, and a ripe avocado for the ultimate nourishing meal. I've lived on this for weeks at a time, proof that healthy eating doesn't need to be complicated – just good food, done right.

Heat the coconut oil in a large pan over a medium heat. Once hot, add the garlic, ginger and chilli. Sauté for 30–60 seconds, stirring frequently, until fragrant and slightly translucent – be careful not to let it burn.

Lower the heat slightly and stir in the turmeric, cumin, coriander, curry powder and garam masala. Cook the spices for about 1–2 minutes, allowing their aroma to deepen.

Pour in the vegetable stock, stirring well to deglaze the pan and combine with the spices. Add the rinsed red lentils and chopped tomatoes, stirring everything together. Reduce the heat to low, cover the pan, and simmer for 20–25 minutes, until the lentils are tender but still holding their shape. Stir occasionally and add a splash of water, if needed.

Stir in the coconut milk and almond butter, and cook uncovered over a low heat for 5 minutes, allowing the flavours to meld.

Season with salt and pepper to taste, stir in the fresh coriander and squeeze in the lemon juice for a final burst of brightness. Serve warm with roasted sweet potatoes, steamed quinoa or rice, leafy greens, avocado and lemon wedges for a nourishing, satisfying meal.

2 tbsp coconut oil

4 garlic cloves, minced

Thumb-sized piece of fresh root ginger, peeled and grated

1 chilli pepper (serrano or jalapeño), finely diced (or 1 tsp cayenne pepper)

1 tbsp grated fresh turmeric (or 1 tsp ground turmeric)

1 tsp ground cumin

1 tsp ground coriander

1 tsp curry powder

1 tsp garam masala

500ml (17fl oz/scant 2¼ cups) vegetable stock

200g (7oz) red lentils, rinsed

1 × 400g (14oz) can chopped tomatoes

250ml (9fl oz/generous 1 cup) full-fat coconut milk

2 tbsp almond butter

Handful of fresh coriander (cilantro), chopped, plus extra to serve

Juice of ½ lemon

Sea salt and black pepper

For Serving (optional)

Roasted sweet potatoes, steamed quinoa or rice

Leafy greens

Sliced avocado

Lemon wedges

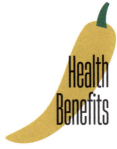

Health Benefits

During World War II, lentils became a staple due to their affordability and high nutritional value, stepping in as a reliable alternative to meat when supplies were scarce. They've been a go-to ever since – not just for their protein content, but for their versatility. From hearty burger patties to plant-based seafood alternatives, lentils do it all. Nutritionally, they're made up of over 25 per cent protein and contain iron, providing around 2mg per 100g (3½oz) cooked – two key nutrients that can sometimes be harder to come by in plant-focused diets.

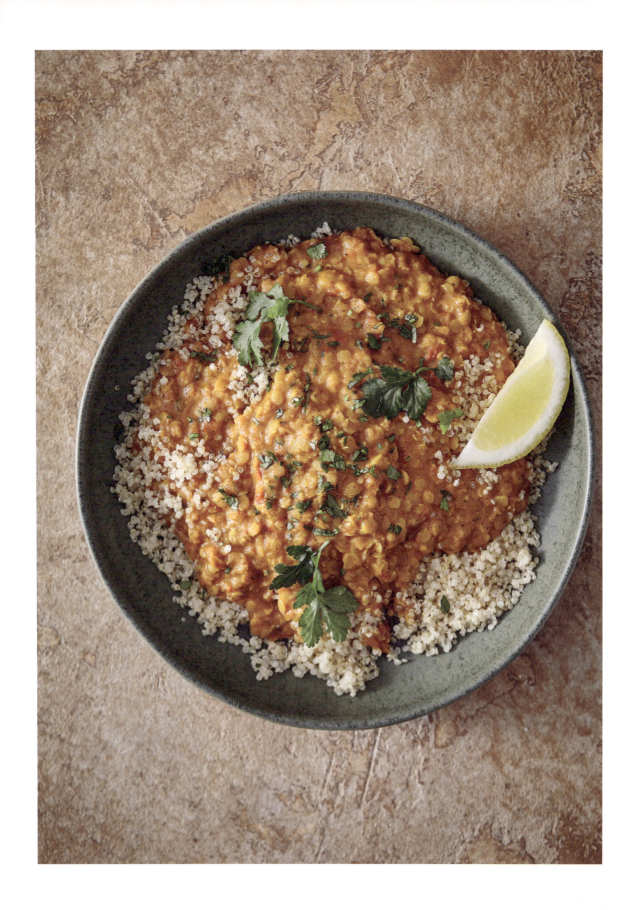

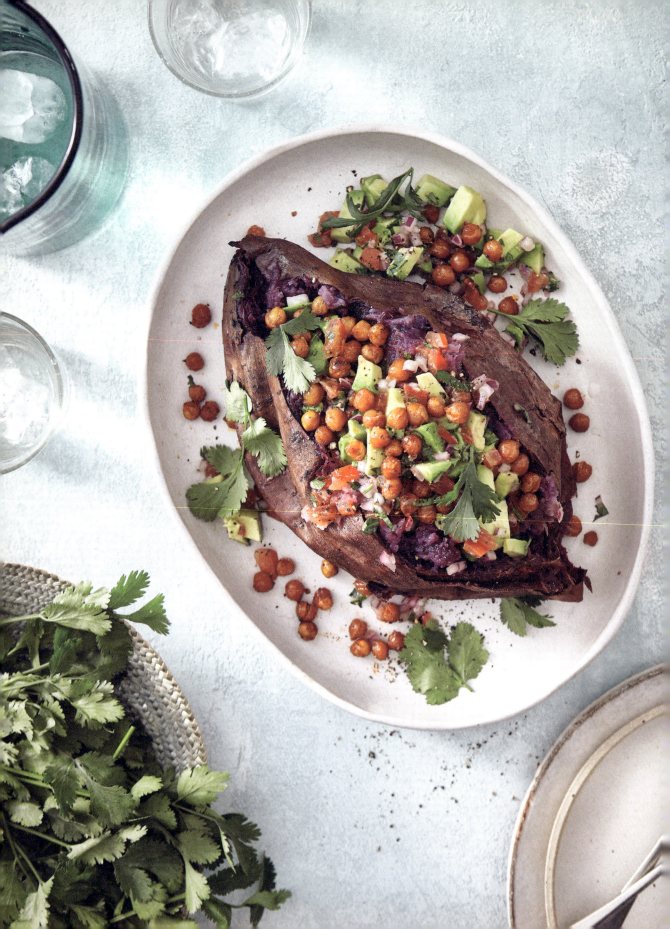

Loaded Sweet Potato

Serves 2
Prep 15 minutes
Cook 45 minutes

Ever wondered what two chefs eat when they come together? Well, I met up with my friend Ramoan (RG Vegan), one of the most creative chefs I know, and this is the dish he made me. I was blown away by how simple yet satisfying and complete it was. Healthy fats, protein, fibre-rich carbs and vibrant veggies – a truly balanced meal that's been on my dinner plate at least once a week ever since.

Preheat the oven to Fan 160°C/180°C/350°F/Gas 4.

Pierce the sweet potatoes with a fork and place them on one side of a baking tray. Spread the drained chickpeas on the other side (or on a separate tray, if needed). Toss the chickpeas with the olive oil, salt, smoked paprika, maple syrup and any optional seasonings. Place the tray in the preheated oven and roast for 20–25 minutes, stirring the chickpeas halfway through, until they are golden and crispy.

Remove the tray from the oven and tip the chickpeas into a serving bowl, leaving them to cool slightly. Return the sweet potatoes to the oven to continue roasting for another 20 minutes, or until tender.

Meanwhile, make the guacamole. In a bowl, mash the avocados with a fork until slightly chunky. Mix in the lime juice, tomato, red onion, garlic, coriander and cayenne pepper, and season with salt to taste.

Slice the roasted sweet potatoes in half and gently mash the insides with a fork to create space for the toppings.

Spoon a generous amount of guacamole onto each sweet potato half, then top with the roasted chickpeas and garnish with fresh coriander. Serve warm with a drizzle of tahini or hot sauce, if desired.

2 large sweet potatoes
1 × 400g (14oz) can chickpeas (garbanzo beans), drained and rinsed
2 tbsp extra-virgin olive oil
½ tsp sea salt
1 tsp smoked paprika
1 tsp maple syrup
¼ tsp ground cumin or cayenne pepper (optional)
Small handful of coriander (cilantro)
Tahini or hot sauce , to serve (optional)

Guacamole

2 ripe avocados, peeled and pitted
Juice of 1 lime
1 small tomato, diced
¼ small red onion, diced
1 garlic clove, minced
1 tbsp freshly chopped coriander (cilantro)
½ tsp cayenne pepper
Sea salt

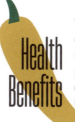

Health Benefits

This dish contains healthy carbohydrates (sweet potato), healthy fats (avocado and olive oil), plant-based protein (chickpeas) and colourful vegetables, making it a balanced and nutritious meal.

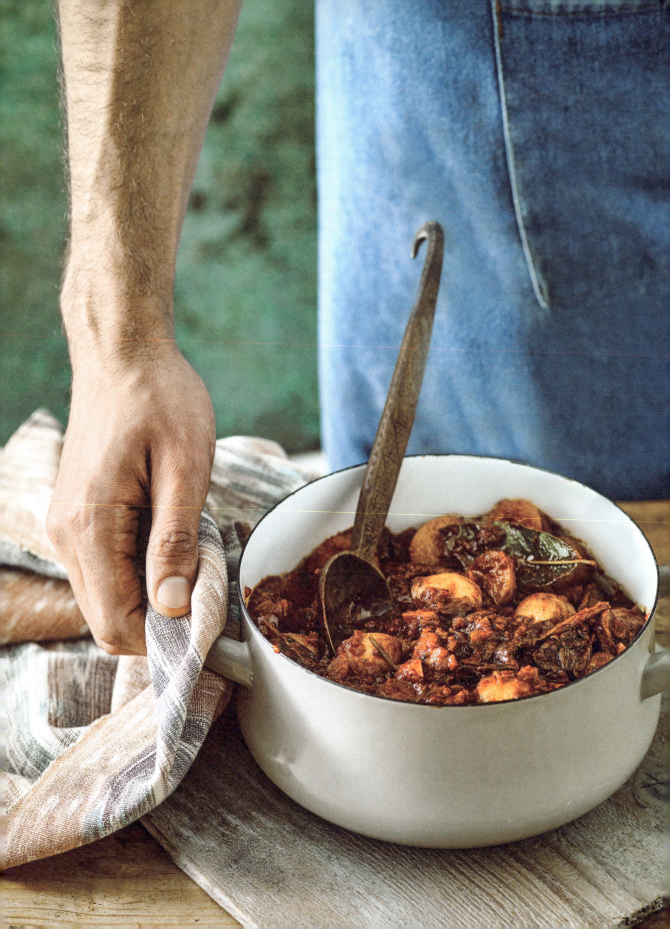

Meaty Mushroom Stew

Serves 3–4
Prep 30 minutes
Cook 1 hour

Mushrooms are one of the most misunderstood foods. The truth is, it's not the mushrooms that people dislike, it's the soggy texture and lack of seasoning. Think about unseasoned, soggy chicken – no one would enjoy that either! Mushrooms have a texture remarkably similar to chicken when prepared correctly. This recipe completely changed how I feel about them. By cooking mushrooms first without oil, you release the excess water, creating a crispier, meatier texture. Once they've absorbed the rich flavours of the stew, you'll never look at mushrooms the same way again. This dish is perfect to share with friends, family, or a loved one, offering comfort that warms the soul and nourishes the spirit.

Heat the olive oil in a large pot over a medium heat. Add the red onion, garlic, cinnamon and allspice, and season with salt and pepper. Cook for 4–5 minutes until the onion is soft and fragrant.

Stir in the spring onions, rosemary, bay leaves and carrots. Let everything cook together for 5–7 minutes, allowing the vegetables to caramelise slightly.

Stir in the date syrup, coating the vegetables, and cook down for 2–3 minutes to add sweetness and depth.

Add the tomato purée and cook for another 2–3 minutes to enhance the flavour.

Pour in the vegetable stock and tomatoes. Stir well to combine. Add the halved potatoes, ensuring there's enough liquid to cover the ingredients. Bring to a boil, then reduce the heat to low, cover with a lid and simmer for 30–40 minutes, or until the potatoes are tender.

While the stew is simmering, season the oyster mushrooms with the onion powder, allspice, smoked paprika, cinnamon, cloves, date syrup and salt.

Place a cast-iron skillet over a medium-high heat. Without adding oil, fry the mushrooms, pressing them down with a spatula to release their moisture. Cook for 5–10 minutes, flipping occasionally, until they are browned, slightly crispy and meaty in texture.

Add the mushrooms to the stew and stir to combine. Leave to simmer for 5 minutes to meld the flavours.

Remove from the heat and set aside for 10–15 minutes to cool slightly and let the flavours fully develop before serving warm.

3 tbsp extra-virgin olive oil
1 large red onion, diced
4 fresh garlic cloves, minced
½ tsp ground cinnamon
1 tsp ground allspice
3 spring onions (scallions), chopped
2 sprigs of rosemary
2 bay leaves
4 carrots, chopped
4 tbsp date syrup
4 tbsp tomato purée (paste)
1 litre (33fl oz/4¼ cups) vegetable stock (or enough to cover the ingredients)
1 × 400g (14oz) can chopped tomatoes
500g (1lb 2oz) baby potatoes, halved
500g (1lb 2oz) oyster mushrooms, torn into large chunks
Sea salt and black pepper

Seasoning for Mushrooms

1 tsp onion powder
½ tsp ground allspice
½ tsp smoked paprika
¼ tsp ground cinnamon
Pinch of ground cloves
2 tbsp date syrup
½ tsp sea salt

Notes

For a unique twist, substitute the potatoes with sweet potatoes to add a touch of sweetness. This stew tastes even better the next day, as the flavours have time to deepen. Store it in an airtight container in the fridge for up to 3 days or freeze it for up to 1 month.

Power Black Bean Stew

Serves 3–4
Prep 7 minutes
Cook 2 hours 10 minutes

Strong, vital and grounded – this is exactly how I feel every time I enjoy this black bean stew. There's something truly special about it. The creamy texture of the black beans, combined with their impressive protein and fibre content, creates a sense of inner strength and warmth that fuels me through the day. That's why I've started calling them Power Beans. This is one of my favourite meals to prep on a Sunday evening for an easy, nourishing and satisfying dinner. Pair it with roasted sweet potato or rice, add some avocado and drizzle with tahini. Pure power on a plate.

Place the olive oil in a large pot over a medium heat. Add the red onion and ginger, and cook for 5–6 minutes, stirring occasionally, until softened and slightly golden.

Stir in the garlic, cumin, cinnamon, oregano, thyme, cayenne pepper and bay leaves. Stir continuously for 1–2 minutes, until the spices are fragrant and well incorporated.

Add the date syrup, tamari and lime juice, and stir thoroughly. Pour in the soaked black beans and vegetable stock, stir to combine, then bring the mixture to a gentle boil. Reduce the heat to low, cover with a lid and simmer gently for 1½–2 hours, until the beans are tender. Stir occasionally, adding more stock or water, if needed, to keep the beans submerged.

Season with salt and remove and discard the bay leaves before serving warm, paired with roasted sweet potatoes or steamed rice and leafy greens. Add a drizzle of tahini and top with sliced avocado and a lime wedge for a creamy, balanced finish, if desired.

4 tbsp extra-virgin olive oil

1 red onion, finely chopped

Thumb-sized piece of fresh root ginger, peeled and grated

4 garlic cloves, minced

1 tsp ground cumin

1 tsp ground cinnamon

1 tbsp dried oregano

1 tbsp dried thyme

1 tsp cayenne pepper

2 bay leaves

3 tbsp date syrup

4 tbsp tamari (or coconut aminos)

Juice of 2 limes

550g (1lb 4oz) dried black beans, soaked for 8–12 hours, then drained (see page 25)

1.5 litres (2¾ pints/6½ cups) vegetable stock

Sea salt

For Serving

Roasted sweet potatoes or steamed rice

Leafy greens (optional)

Tahini (optional)

Sliced avocado (optional)

Lime wedges (optional)

Notes

This stew develops even richer flavours when reheated. Store leftovers in an airtight container in the fridge for up to 5 days or freeze for up to 3 months.

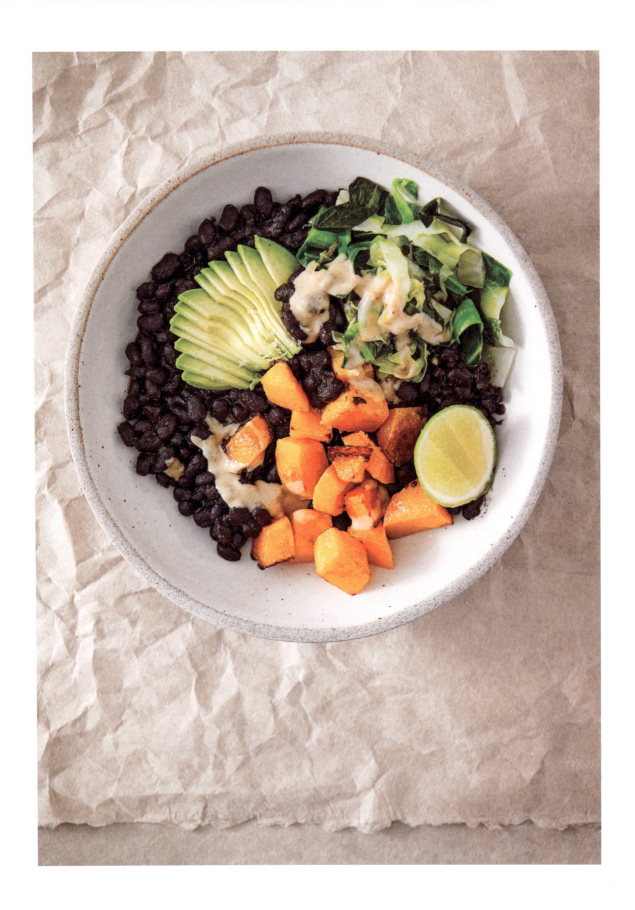

Tofu Bolognese

This was my first-ever home-cooked meal using only unprocessed ingredients and, to this day, it's still one I recommend to anyone transitioning to a whole-foods diet. If you're still not convinced that eating natural, whole foods can be both satisfying and nourishing, I highly suggest you try it. It's the Bolognese that foodie dreams are made of – rich and hearty, using ingredients that serve your body well, leaving you full, but not bloated. If is satisfying, but not greasy, and nourishing, but not heavy. What more could you ask for?

Using a fork, crumble the tofu into small pieces until it resembles minced (ground) meat.

Heat the olive oil in a large skillet or frying pan over a medium heat. Add the crumbled tofu and fry for about 5 minutes, stirring frequently, until crispy and golden.

Stir in the chopped onion and garlic, and cook for 2 minutes until softened.

Add the tomato purée, stir well, and cook for another 2 minutes to enhance the flavours.

Stir in the date syrup and mix thoroughly. Add the puréed tomatoes, maple syrup and oregano. Stir to combine and let the sauce simmer for 3 minutes. Season with salt and pepper to taste.

Meanwhile, cook the pasta in boiling salted water according to the packet instructions until al dente. Drain and set aside.

Stir the chopped basil into the sauce just before serving.

Divide the pasta and Bolognese between 2–3 plates, and top with the toasted pine nuts and more basil leaves, to serve.

250g (9oz) firm tofu
3½ tbsp extra-virgin olive oil
1 red onion, finely chopped
2 garlic cloves, minced
4 tbsp tomato purée (paste)
3 tbsp date syrup
150g (5½oz) puréed tomatoes or passata
1–2 tbsp maple syrup
1 tsp dried oregano
250g (9oz) pasta (spelt or buckwheat preferrably)
Small bunch of basil leaves, chopped, plus extra whole leaves to serve
50g (1¾oz) pine nuts, toasted
Sea salt and black pepper

Notes

Spelt pasta works wonderfully in this recipe, offering a hearty texture and flavour. For a gluten-free alternative, opt for buckwheat or lentil pasta. These options are more satiating and nutrient-dense than standard pasta.

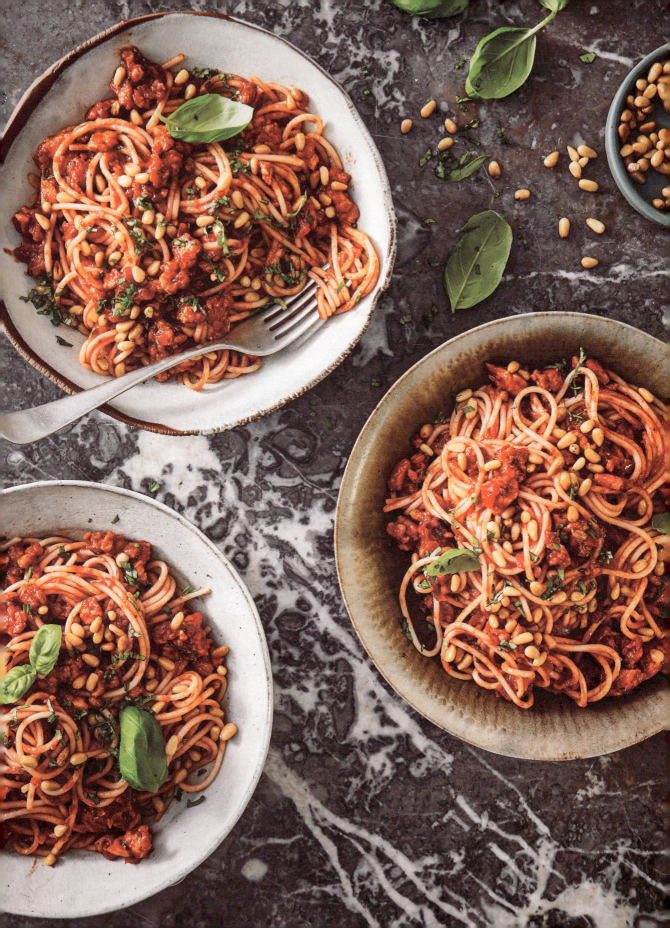

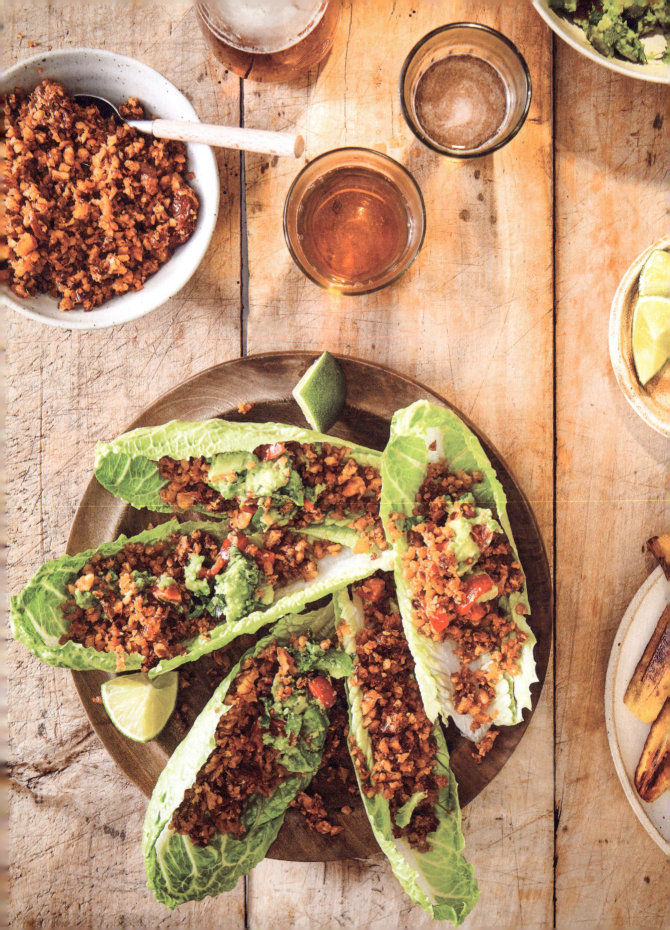

Walnut 'Meat'

I still remember the first time I made this dish – it was one of those days when I wanted something hearty and satisfying, but unprocessed. I opened my pantry, saw a bag of walnuts and thought, 'What can I do with these?' Fast forward and now this walnut 'meat' has become a staple in my kitchen. It's not just about the flavour (which is incredible), it's the idea that these humble, brain-shaped nuts are feeding both body and mind. Every bite feels nourishing, grounding and full of purpose. Real food for thought.

Place the soaked walnuts in a food processor and pulse until they resemble coarse crumbs. Be careful not to overdo it – you want a 'meaty' texture.

Heat the olive oil in a large skillet or frying pan over a medium heat. Toss in the onion and sauté for about 2–3 minutes, until soft and translucent.

Add the garlic and cook for 1 minute, stirring frequently to prevent burning.

Sprinkle in the cayenne pepper, smoked paprika, allspice and salt, stirring well to coat the onion and garlic. Let the spices bloom in the heat for about 30 seconds, then add the sun-dried tomatoes and cook for 1 minute, stirring to combine.

Add the crumbled walnuts and stir well to ensure they soak up all the flavours.

Pour in the lime juice and date or maple syrup, stirring thoroughly. Cook for another 4–5 minutes, stirring occasionally, until the mixture is heated through and well combined. If the mixture starts to feel dry, add a tablespoon of water or a drizzle of more oil.

Remove from the heat and serve the walnut meat in romaine lettuce leaves as wraps, or pair with guacamole, quinoa or plantains, and lime wedges.

275g (9¾oz) walnuts, soaked for 4–6 hours, then drained (see page 25)
2–3 tbsp extra-virgin olive oil
1 red onion, finely chopped
4 garlic cloves, minced
½ tsp cayenne pepper
1 tsp smoked paprika
1 tsp ground allspice
1 tsp sea salt
30g (1oz) sun-dried tomatoes in oil, finely chopped
Juice of 1 lime
2 tbsp date syrup or maple syrup

For Serving (optional)
Romaine lettuce
Guacamole (see page 99)
Steamed quinoa
Plantain
Lime wedges

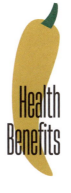

Health Benefits

The ancient Doctrine of Signatures teaches us that foods often resemble the parts of the body they nourish. Walnuts are high in manganese which is important for brain function and also regulates nerve impulse progression.

Butternut Bean Curry

One rainy autumn afternoon, I made my favourite pumpkin soup. I wondered if there was a way to add a good source of protein to it. Then I spotted a jar of butterbeans in my cupboard. Their neutral taste and creamy texture had me hooked. To this day, not many dishes compare when I want something warming, yet complete.

Preheat the oven to Fan 210°C/230°C/450°F/Gas 8 and line a baking tray with parchment paper.

Pierce the squash a few times with a knife or fork. Coat it lightly with some of the olive oil, then place it on the prepared baking tray and roast in the preheated oven for 30–35 minutes or until tender. Leave it to cool for about 15 minutes, then peel off the skin and scoop out the flesh, discarding the seeds.

Put the roasted squash and coconut milk in a high-speed blender or food processor and blend until smooth and creamy. Set aside.

Heat the remaining olive oil in a large pan over a medium heat. Add the onion and sauté for 4–5 minutes, until soft and translucent. Stir in the garlic, ginger, cinnamon, turmeric and smoked paprika. Cook for 1–2 minutes, stirring frequently, until the spices are fragrant. Add the butter beans to the pan and stir well to coat them in the spices and aromatics. Cook for 3–4 minutes to allow the beans to absorb the flavours.

Pour the squash and coconut mixture into the pan and stir until well combined. Reduce the heat to low, cover with a lid and simmer gently for 10 minutes, stirring occasionally, until the sauce thickens slightly and the flavours meld.

Remove the pan from the heat, stir in the lemon juice and season to taste. Sprinkle over the fresh coriander and serve in warm bowls.

1 medium butternut squash
2–3 tbsp extra-virgin olive oil
360ml (12fl oz/1½ cups) coconut milk
1 brown onion, diced
3 garlic cloves, minced
1 tsp finely grated fresh root ginger
½ tsp ground cinnamon
½ tsp ground turmeric
½ tsp smoked paprika
2 × 400g (14oz) cans butter (lima) beans, drained and rinsed
Juice of 1 lemon
Handful of fresh coriander (cilantro), chopped
Sea salt and black pepper

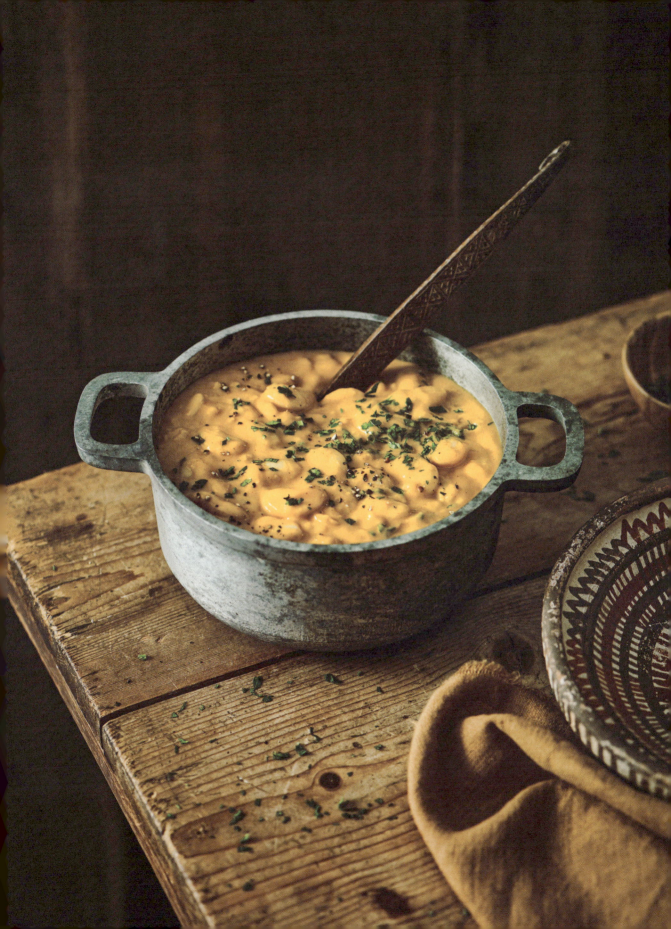

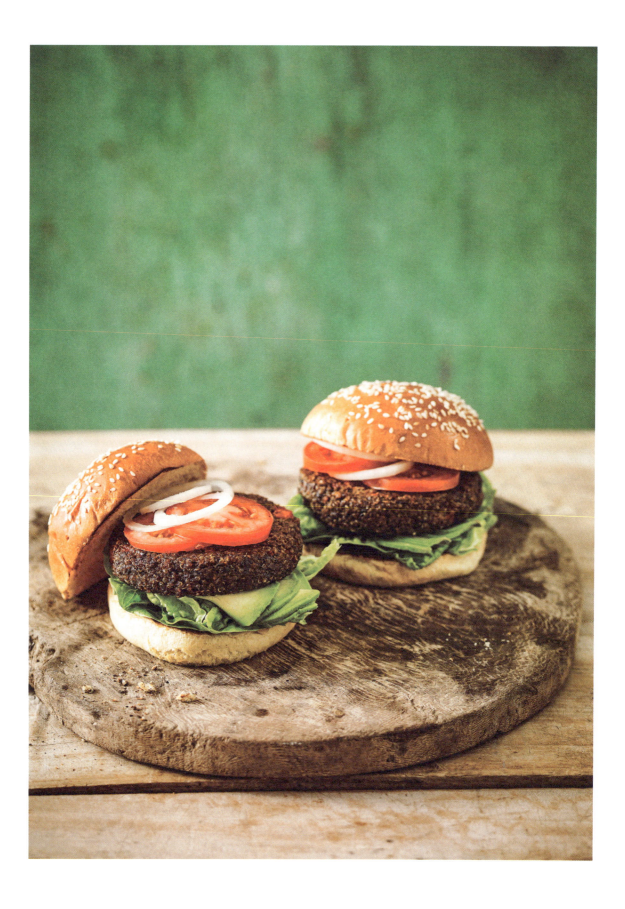

Black Bean Power Burger

This isn't just any old veggie burger – it's a power burger, built from a trio of ingredients that bring more than just flavour: black beans for strength, quinoa for grounded energy, and mushrooms for vitality. Together they create a burger that's smoky, hearty and packed with real sustenance. The spices do the heavy lifting, bringing warmth and depth, while the texture is spot-on – crispy on the outside, soft but structured on the inside. Serve it in a bun, in a bowl, or on its own. However you plate it, this is fuel.

Preheat the oven to Fan 180°C/200°C/400°F/Gas 6.

Place a pan over a medium heat. Add the oil, onion, garlic and bell pepper, and sauté for 5–7 minutes until soft and caramelised – don't let it burn. Stir in the onion powder, allspice, cayenne pepper and smoked paprika, and cook for 1 minute to release the flavours. Remove from heat and set aside to cool slightly.

Toss the mushrooms with a little olive oil, and season with salt and pepper. Place them on a baking tray and roast in the preheated oven for 15–20 minutes, until tender and slightly browned.

Meanwhile, place the quinoa in a pot with 260ml (9fl oz/generous 1 cup) water. Bring to a boil, then lower the heat and simmer for 10–15 minutes until fluffy. Set aside to cool.

In a food processor or high-speed blender, combine the sautéed onions, garlic and bell pepper, the roasted mushrooms, cooked quinoa, black beans, flour, arrowroot, if using, and date or maple syrup, and season with salt and pepper. Pulse until the mixture is well combined but still has some texture.

Transfer the mixture to a bowl and leave at room temperature for 30 minutes, or chill in the fridge to firm up – this step helps everything bind properly.

Shape the mixture into 4–5 burger patties, then place them in the fridge for another 15–30 minutes to firm. The colder they are, the better they'll hold their shape when cooking.

Place a frying pan over a medium heat, add a little neutral oil and fry the patties for 3–5 minutes on each side, until golden brown and crisp on the outside.

Assemble in a burger bun with your favourite toppings, or go bunless and serve with salad, avocado and roasted vegetables.

2 tbsp avocado oil or extra-virgin olive oil, plus extra to drizzle

1 red onion, finely diced

3 garlic cloves, minced

1 red bell pepper, deseeded and sliced

1 tsp onion powder

1 tsp ground allspice

½ tsp cayenne pepper

2 tsp smoked paprika

160g (5¾oz) mushrooms (oyster, chestnut/cremini, or button)

130g (4½oz) quinoa, rinsed

1 × 400g (14oz) can black beans, drained and rinsed

2–3 tbsp spelt flour (buckwheat or chickpea flour for a gluten-free option)

1 tsp arrowroot powder (for better binding)

2 tbsp date syrup (or 1 tsp maple syrup)

Neutral oil, for frying

Sea salt and black pepper

For Serving (optional)

4–5 burger buns

Salad

Avocado

Roasted vegetables

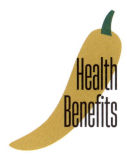

Health Benefits

Black beans bring protein, fibre and folic acid, making them a brilliant nutrient-dense legume. Quinoa is a complete protein, meaning it provides all nine essential amino acids, while mushrooms add a range of vitamins and rich umami depth. This burger isn't about imitating – it's about celebrating real ingredients that work together to nourish, satisfy and keep you powered up.

Chilli

The ultimate meal-prep recipe – just double or triple the quantities for an easy fix. With simple ingredients, nutrient-dense components and quick prep, it's perfect for batch cooking – and it tastes even better the following day. I like to prepare a big batch on Sunday evening, then all I have to do during the week is reheat a portion, slice up some avocado and spring onions, and serve. It is also a great dish to prepare for your friends.

Using a fork or your hands, crumble the firm tofu into very small pieces.

Heat the olive oil in a large skillet or pan over a medium heat. Add the crumbled tofu and fry for about 5 minutes, stirring occasionally, until lightly golden.

Stir in the chopped onions and cook for another 5 minutes, until softened and fragrant.

Add the tomato purée and maple syrup, stir well, and cook for about 2 minutes, allowing the mixture to caramelise slightly.

Stir in the puréed tomatoes, kidney beans, sweetcorn, oregano, cumin and chilli, and season with salt and pepper. Mix everything thoroughly. Cook for another 2–3 minutes, allowing the flavours to meld and the mixture to thicken slightly.

Serve hot with quinoa or tortilla chips for dipping, and garnish with sliced spring onions, sliced avocado and lime wedges, if you like.

200g (7oz) firm tofu

3½ tbsp extra-virgin olive oil

2 brown onions, finely chopped

200g (7oz) tomato purée (paste)

3 tbsp maple syrup

330ml (11fl oz) puréed tomatoes

170g (6oz) kidney beans, drained and rinsed

130g (4½oz) sweetcorn

1 tbsp dried oregano

½ tbsp ground cumin

½ Scotch bonnet chilli or 1 tsp cayenne pepper (adjust to taste)

Sea salt and black pepper

For Serving (optional)

Steamed quinoa or tortilla chips

Finely sliced spring onion (scallion)

Sliced avocado

Lime wedges

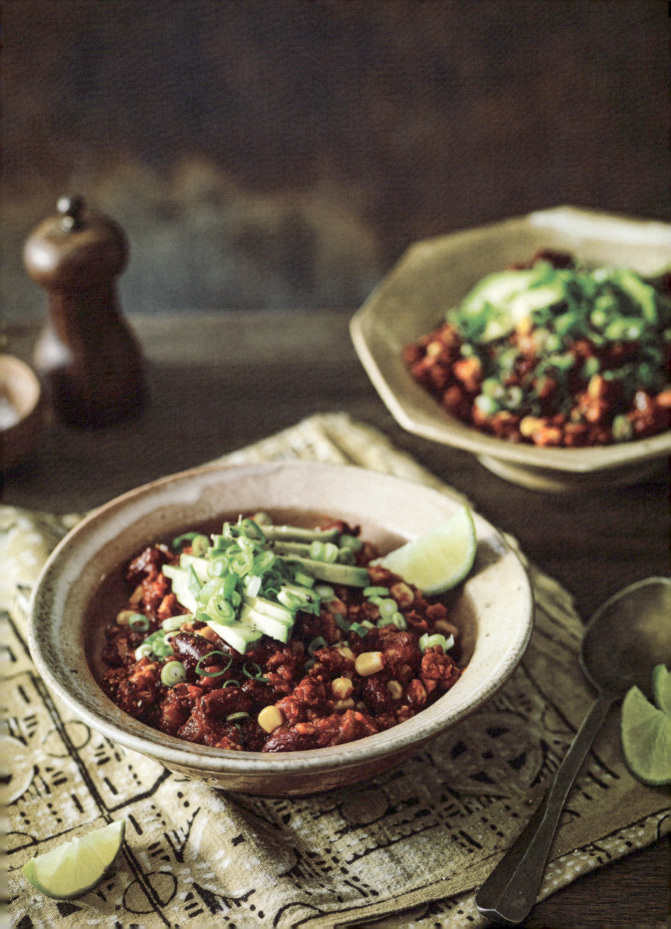

Comforting Chickpea Noodle Soup

Serves 3–4
Prep 10 minutes
Cook 22 minutes

In many traditional medicine systems, foods are classified by their energetic properties – warming or cooling – and, with the right knowledge, you can use their energetic properties to restore balance within the body. This noodle soup is packed with warming ingredients, like turmeric and cayenne pepper, making it feel like a comforting hug for the soul. It's the perfect remedy when you're feeling drained or in need of extra warmth for your heart and spirit. Plus, it's a clever way to incorporate nutrient-rich vegetables, like celery, blending their benefits seamlessly into the dish without overpowering the flavour.

Heat the oil in a large pot over a medium-high heat. Add the diced onion, carrots and celery, and cook for 5–6 minutes, stirring occasionally, until the onion becomes soft and translucent.

Pour in the vegetable stock, then stir in the onion powder, garlic powder, turmeric, cayenne pepper, oregano, spring onions and chickpeas. Add the pasta and bring the soup to a gentle boil. Reduce the heat to a simmer and cook for 12–15 minutes, or until the pasta and vegetables are tender. Stir occasionally to prevent the pasta from sticking.

Stir in the chopped parsley and season with salt and pepper to taste before serving.

2 tbsp extra-virgin olive oil or avocado oil

1 small brown onion, diced

2 carrots, peeled and diced

3 celery stalks, diced

2 litres (4¼ pints/8¾ cups) vegetable stock

2 tsp onion powder

1 tsp garlic powder

½ tsp ground turmeric

1 tsp cayenne pepper

1 tsp dried oregano

2 spring onions (scallions), finely sliced

1 × 400g (14oz) can chickpeas (garbanzo beans), drained and rinsed

225g (8oz) spelt, buckwheat or lentil pasta

15g (½oz) fresh parsley, chopped

Sea salt and black pepper

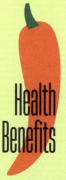

Health Benefits

This hearty soup is a perfect warming dish for cold winter days, offering comfort and nourishment in every spoonful. With its blend of protein-rich chickpeas (garbanzo beans), vibrant vegetables and warming spices, this soup not only satisfies but also provides essential nutrients to keep you energised during the colder months.

Chickpea Curry

Serves 2–3
Prep 10 minutes
Cook 35 minutes

When I first visited Jamaica, I stayed on a farm with a man named Bobby, who introduced me to Rastafari – a religious and social movement – and the Ital lifestyle, which emphasises eating foods grown from the earth, fostering a deeper connection with nature and promoting mindful eating. One of the dishes Bobby taught me was this chickpea curry and, to this day, it's one of my most frequently recreated recipes. It's perfect for meal prepping and pairs beautifully with boiled sweet potato, leafy greens and avocado. Eat to thrive!

Place a pot over a medium heat and add the oil and the red onion. Sauté for 4–5 minutes until softened.

Stir in the garlic, ginger and dates, and sauté for 1–2 minutes, until fragrant.

Sprinkle in the turmeric, cinnamon, ground cloves, cumin, onion powder, cayenne pepper, salt and pepper. Cook for 2 minutes to toast the spices and release their aroma.

Pour in the chickpeas, coconut milk and maple syrup and stir well to combine. Bring to a boil, then reduce the heat to low, cover with a lid and simmer gently for 20–25 minutes, stirring occasionally to prevent sticking.

Remove from the heat and squeeze in the lime juice.

Serve hot, garnished with spring onions, if using, and alongside rice or sweet potato, and avocado for a complete meal.

2 tbsp extra-virgin olive oil

1 red onion, chopped

3 garlic cloves, minced

Thumb-sized piece of fresh root ginger, peeled and grated

2–3 medjool dates, pitted and chopped

1 tsp ground turmeric

1 tsp ground cinnamon

½ tsp ground cloves

1 tsp ground cumin

1 tbsp onion powder

1 tsp cayenne pepper

1 tsp sea salt

Pinch of black pepper

320g (11½ oz) cooked chickpeas (garbanzo beans)

500ml (18fl oz/generous 2 cups) coconut milk

1 tsp maple syrup

Juice of 1 lime

For Serving

Small bunch of spring onions (scallions), sliced (optional)

Steamed rice or sweet potato

1 avocado, sliced

Notes

This curry is perfect for meal prepping – just double the quantities. Store portions in airtight containers and keep in the fridge for up to 3 days or freeze for up to 1 month.

Rustic Tuscan Bean & Kale Soup

Serves 4–5
Prep 15 minutes
Cook 25 minutes

There's something about a pot of soup simmering away that just feels right. It's simple, wholesome and always greater than the sum of its parts. This one is a favourite – creamy cannellini beans, soft potatoes and fragrant herbs, all coming together in a way that just works. Blending part of it gives it that perfectly thick, velvety texture while keeping enough bite to make it feel hearty. Stir in some fresh kale at the end, drizzle over good olive oil, squeeze in some lemon and you've got a bowl that's just as nourishing as it is satisfying.

Heat the olive oil in a large pot over a medium heat. Add the onion, celery and carrots and a pinch of salt, and sauté for about 3–5 minutes, stirring occasionally, until the vegetables start to soften.

Stir in the garlic and cayenne pepper and cook for 1 minute, letting the spices bloom and the garlic turn fragrant.

Pour in the vegetable stock, scraping up any bits from the bottom of the pot to bring out extra flavour. Add the beans, potatoes, rosemary, sage and bay leaves, and season with salt and pepper. Stir well and bring to a gentle boil. Reduce the heat, cover with a lid and simmer for 15 minutes, or until the potatoes are tender.

Remove the bay leaves, rosemary and sage, then transfer about half of the soup to a food processor (or use a stick blender) to blitz until smooth and creamy. Return to the pot and stir well.

Add the kale to the soup and cook over a low heat for 3–5 minutes, until just wilted and tender.

Ladle into bowls and finish with a drizzle of extra-virgin olive oil and a squeeze of lemon juice to bring out the flavours.

2 tbsp extra-virgin olive oil, plus extra for drizzling

1 large brown onion, diced

3 celery stalks, diced

3 carrots, peeled and diced

5 garlic cloves, minced

½ tsp cayenne pepper

1½ litres (3¼ pints/6½ cups) vegetable stock

1 × 400g (14oz) can cannellini beans (or butter/lima beans), drained and rinsed

2 large potatoes, diced

1 sprig of fresh rosemary (or 2 tsp dried)

1 sprig of fresh sage (or 2 tsp dried)

2 bay leaves

100g (3½oz) kale, stalks removed and leaves chopped

Juice of ½ lemon

Sea salt and black pepper

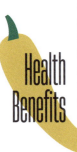

Health Benefits

This soup is packed with fibre, protein, vitamins and minerals from the beans, potatoes and kale – keeping you full and fuelling your body with slow-burning energy. Cannellini beans are rich in plant-based protein and fibre, while kale delivers a hit of chlorophyll and essential vitamins. The herbs don't just add flavour, they're packed with nutrients and naturally occuring chemicals that could help nourish the gut microbiome and may help decrease chronic inflammation.

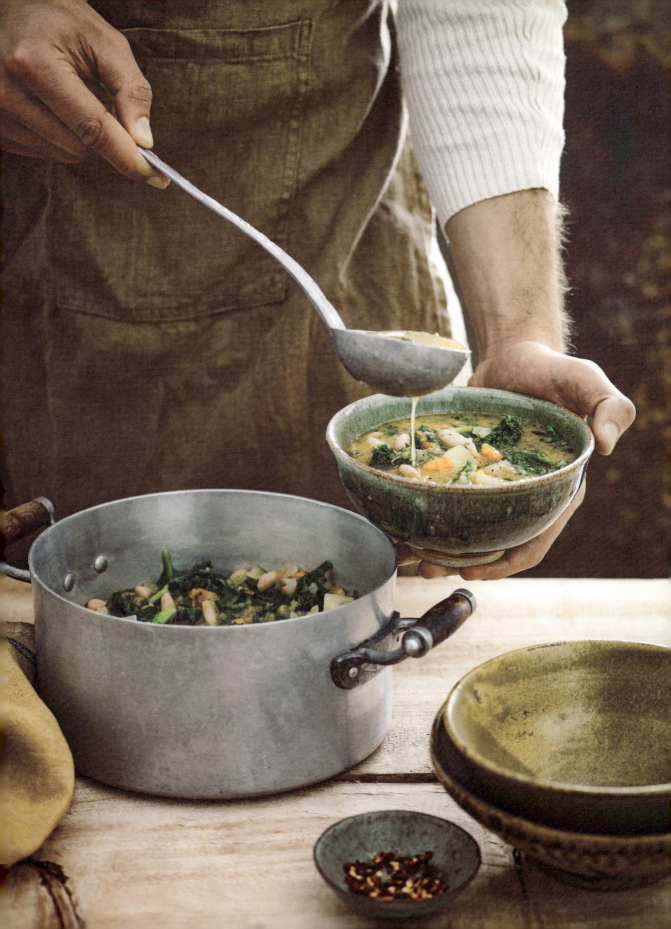

The Lentil Stew You Won't Forget

Serves 2–4
Prep 10 minutes
Cook 45 minutes

Some meals make you realise you're missing absolutely nothing by eating unprocessed, whole foods. This is one of them. The first time I made this dish, I knew it had to be shared with the world. The deep, slow-simmered spices, the richness of the caramelised onions, and the way the lentils soaked up every drop of flavour – it was the kind of meal that didn't just satisfy hunger but left an impression. This isn't just food; it's a warm, bold and nourishing experience.

Heat the oil in a large pot over a medium heat. Add the red onion, spring onions, ginger and garlic, season with a pinch of salt, and sauté for 3–4 minutes until fragrant.

Stir in the allspice, onion powder, thyme, cayenne, nutmeg and cinnamon, letting the spices toast for a couple of minutes.

Add the tomatoes and cook for 5–7 minutes, stirring occasionally, until they break down and become saucy.

Stir in the lentils, vegetable stock, date syrup (or maple syrup), and another pinch of salt and pepper. Stir well and bring to a boil. Reduce the heat, cover with a lid and simmer for 25–30 minutes, stirring occasionally, until the lentils are soft and most of the liquid is absorbed. Set aside for a couple of minutes before serving.

This is perfect with rice, plantains, or fresh greens.

2 tbsp extra-virgin olive oil or avocado oil
1 red onion, finely chopped
3 spring onions (scallions), finely sliced
Thumb-sized piece of fresh root ginger, peeled and grated
4–5 garlic cloves, minced
1 tsp ground allspice
1 tsp onion powder
1 tsp dried thyme
1 tsp cayenne pepper (adjust to taste)
½ tsp ground nutmeg
½ tsp ground cinnamon
3 large tomatoes, finely chopped
200g (7oz/1 cup) brown lentils, rinsed
500ml (18fl oz/scant 2¼ cups) vegetable stock
2 tbsp date syrup (or 1 tbsp maple syrup)
Sea salt and black pepper

For Serving
Steamed rice, plantains or fresh greens

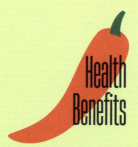

Health Benefits

Lentils are a top-tier, plant-based protein source, packed with fibre, selenium, folic acid and slow-burning energy. The mix of warming spices, like allspice, nutmeg, cinnamon, ginger and cayenne not only enhance the depth of flavour, but also increase the range of natural planted-based chemicals.

One-Pot Quinoa Chickpea Meal

Serves 2
Prep 5 minutes
Cook 45 minutes

This is one of my meal-prep favourites. And the best part? Everything can be prepared in one pot. Simple, yet effective – that's what I'm all about when it comes to busy weekdays. I want something nourishing, without breaking the bank or spending hours cooking and cleaning countless dishes. I love prepping this and storing it in containers in the fridge, so when I get home tired, I have a healthy, wholesome dinner waiting for me.

To make the spiced chickpeas, heat the extra-virgin olive oil in a large skillet or frying pan over a medium heat. Add the chickpeas and fry for 4–5 minutes, stirring occasionally, until golden and crispy. Sprinkle with cayenne pepper, onion powder, smoked paprika and salt, and cook for another 3–4 minutes, allowing the chickpeas to absorb the spices. Transfer to a plate and set aside.

Using the same skillet or pan, make the quinoa base. Add the extra-virgin olive oil, chopped onion and salt, and cook over a medium heat for 4–5 minutes until the onion softens and caramelises.

Reduce the heat to medium-low, stir in the chopped ginger, and fry for 2–3 minutes.

Add the passata, stirring well, and cook for 2 minutes.

Add the rinsed quinoa, along with the basil, oregano, onion powder and allspice. Stir well to coat the quinoa in all the flavours. Pour in 360ml (12fl oz/ 1½ cups) water and increase the heat to bring to a boil. Reduce the heat, cover with a lid and simmer for 20–25 minutes, or until the quinoa has absorbed the liquid.

Fold in the crispy chickpeas and all the toppings. Mix well to combine and serve warm.

Spiced Chickpeas

1 tbsp extra-virgin olive oil
240g (8½oz) cooked chickpeas (garbanzo beans)
1 tsp cayenne pepper
1 tsp onion powder
½ tsp smoked paprika
½ tsp sea salt

Quinoa Base

2 tbsp extra-virgin olive oil
80g (2¾oz) brown onion, chopped
½ tsp sea salt
1 tbsp finely grated fresh root ginger
180ml (6fl oz) passata
170g (6oz) uncooked quinoa, rinsed
1 tsp dried basil
1 tsp dried oregano
1 tsp onion powder
½ tsp ground allspice

Toppings

15g (½oz) fresh coriander (cilantro), chopped
50g (1¾oz) sun-dried tomatoes, chopped
30g (1oz) raisins or dates, finely chopped

RESTORE

119

SAUCES, SPREADS & SIDES

ENHANCE

Healthy Yeast-Free Flat Bread

No yeast, no baking powder, no additives - just simple, real ingredients coming together to create the perfect soft, slightly chewy flatbread. Spelt – an ancient grain that's stood the test of time – was once a staple for Ancient Egyptians and even Roman gladiators, who relied on it for strength and endurance. Naturally rich in fibre and nutrients, it makes these flatbreads not just satisfying but deeply nourishing. The coconut yoghurt adds richness, and the sparkling water keeps the dough light and airy, all without needing a single leavening agent. Wrap it, dip it, or load it up – this one works with everything.

3 garlic cloves, minced

2 tsp sea salt

3 tbsp extra-virgin olive oil, plus extra for drizzling

65g (2¼oz/heaped ¼ cup) coconut yoghurt

5 tbsp sparkling water

275g (9¾oz/2 cups) spelt flour, plus extra for dusting

In a bowl, mix the garlic, salt, olive oil, coconut yoghurt and sparkling water until well combined.

Add the spelt flour to a large mixing bowl and create a well in the centre. Pour in the wet ingredients and start mixing with a wooden spoon until a rough dough forms.

Lightly dust a clean work surface with flour. Transfer the dough to the surface and knead for a few minutes until it becomes smooth and elastic.

Divide the dough into eight equal portions. Shape each piece into a ball, flatten slightly with the palm of your hand, then dust both sides with a little flour. Using a rolling pin, roll out each dough ball into a thin, round flatbread (about 12–15cm/4½–6in in diameter).

Place a dry frying pan over a medium heat. When hot, add a flatbread and cook for 2–3 minutes on each side, until golden spots appear and it puffs up slightly. Stack the cooked flatbreads on a plate and cover with a clean tea towel to keep them warm and soft. Repeat with the remaining dough.

Serve the flatbreads warm and drizzle with some extra-virgin olive oil.

Notes

Flour swaps – if you don't have spelt flour, you can use wholemeal plain flour instead. The texture will still be soft and pliable, with a slightly nuttier taste. Why coconut yoghurt? The natural acidity of coconut yoghurt helps to keep the dough soft and tender, adding a slight richness without overpowering the flavour. What's the deal with sparkling water? Instead of relying on yeast or baking powder, the bubbles in sparkling water create a light, soft dough, aerating it for the perfect texture.

Clockwise from top left
Pea Mint, Carrot, Chickpea Tomato and Chive Tofu spreads.

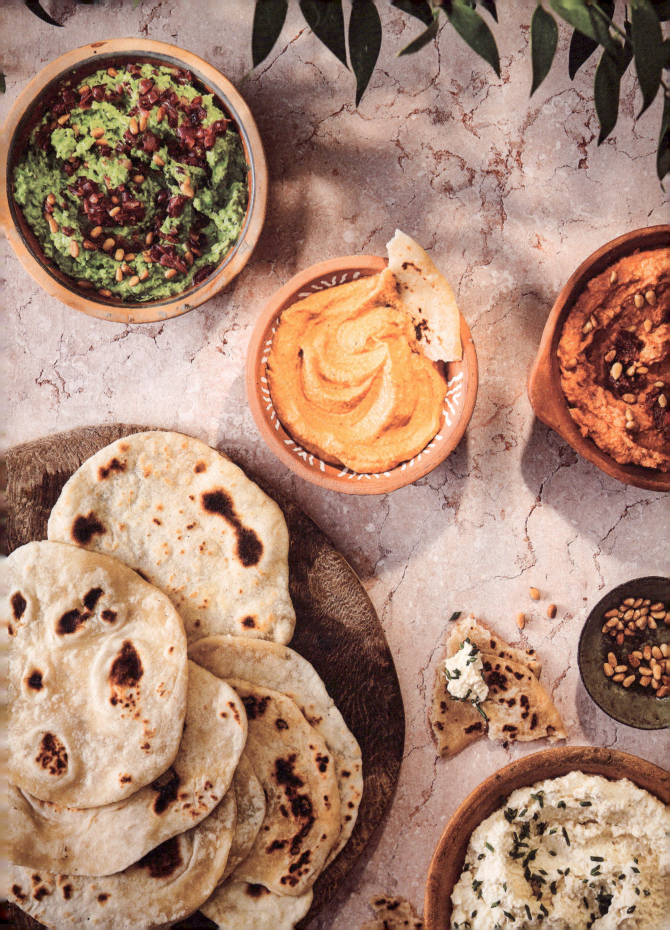

Pea Mint Spread

Serves 6–8
Prep 5 minutes
Cook 13 minutes

I believe the reason many vegetables are disliked today is because of how they're prepared. From mushrooms to aubergines and peas, they often don't get the love they deserve. Peas, in particular, are one of the most versatile foods around. When used right, they're a true delight for the tastebuds. Their creamy texture makes them the perfect base for a spread, similar to using chickpeas in hummus but packed with the nutrients of vibrant green veg. Blend them with pine nuts, onions, mint and olive oil, and you've got a new favourite spread in minutes. Who says healthy eating has to be complicated?

250g (9oz) frozen peas
50g (1¾oz) pine nuts
7 tbsp extra-virgin olive oil
1 small red onion, finely diced

15–20g (½–¾oz) fresh mint, finely chopped
Sea salt and black pepper
Soughdough bread, toasted

Bring a pot of water to a boil and add the frozen peas. Cook for 6–7 minutes, until tender, then drain and set aside.

In a dry skillet or frying pan over a medium heat, toast the pine nuts for 2–3 minutes, stirring frequently, until golden brown and fragrant. Remove from the heat and set aside.

Heat 2 tablespoons of the olive oil in a frying pan over a medium heat. Add the onion and cook for 2–3 minutes until lightly browned and softened. Set aside.

In a high-speed blender or food processor, combine the cooked peas, fresh mint, remaining olive oil and a pinch of salt and pepper. Blend until smooth. Adjust seasoning to taste.

Transfer the mixture to a bowl and stir in the toasted pine nuts and sautéed onions until evenly incorporated.

Serve on toasted sourdough bread.

Carrot Spread

Serves 6–8
Prep 5 minutes

If you're not a fan of attracting unwanted attention, this spread might not be for you – because it steals the spotlight every time. Whether at a breakfast gathering or friends stopping by, it effortlessly becomes the highlight. With simple ingredients you likely already have at home, it doesn't seem a likely star of the show, but one taste is all it takes to understand the hype. The natural sweetness of carrots and tomato purée, combined with the creamy richness of cashews, creates something truly magical. A must-try.

1 shallot, finely diced
50g (1¾oz) cashews, soaked for 2–4 hours, then drained (see page 25)
250g (9oz) carrots, chopped
120g (4¼oz) tomato purée (paste)
1 tsp dried thyme

1 tsp dried oregano
1 tsp sea salt
1 tbsp maple syrup
Soughdough bread, toasted, to serve (optional)
Fresh vegetables, to serve (optional)

In a high-speed blender or food processor, combine all the ingredients and blend until smooth, stopping to scrape down the sides, as needed, to ensure an even consistency.

Serve immediately, or chill in the fridge for a few hours. Enjoy on toasted sourdough, as a sandwich filling, or as a dip for fresh vegetables.

Chickpea Tomato Spread

Serves 6–8
Prep 5 minutes

You might have noticed a common theme throughout this book: nearly every recipe – whether it's a side, smoothie, breakfast, or dip – can stand on its own as a complete, balanced meal. Packed with protein, fibre, healthy fats and colourful veg, these dishes are as satisfying as they are nourishing. So, if you find yourself enjoying this chickpea tomato spread with a fresh baguette for dinner, rest assured, it's as nutritionally complete as it is irresistible. And, trust me, once you get a taste, you won't even think about reaching for anything else!

200g (7oz) cooked chickpeas (garbanzo beans)
60g (2¼oz) sun-dried tomatoes
2 garlic cloves, peeled
60g (2¼oz) tahini
3 tbsp fresh lemon juice
3 tbsp extra-virgin olive oil, plus extra to garnish
1 tsp dried oregano
½–1 tsp sea salt, to taste
Pinch of black pepper
Small handful of pine nuts, toasted, to garnish (optional)
Fresh bread or crackers, to serve (optional)
Fresh vegetables, to serve (optional)

In a high-speed blender or food processor, combine the chickpeas, sun-dried tomatoes, garlic, tahini, lemon juice, olive oil, oregano, salt and a pinch of pepper. Blend until smooth, scraping down the sides as needed. If the mixture is too thick, add a few tablespoons of water or olive oil to achieve your desired consistency.

Taste and adjust the seasoning, adding more salt or lemon juice, if needed.

Transfer the spread to a serving dish. Garnish with toasted pine nuts, if using, and a drizzle of olive oil. This pairs beautifully with fresh bread, crackers or vegetable sticks.

Chive Tofu Spread

Serves 6–8
Prep 3 minutes

If you're looking to build muscle on a plant-focused diet, it's crucial to make every ingredient count. That's why I recreated a classic cheese spread, swapping out the dairy for tofu and cashews. The healthy fats and amino acids give your body what it needs to support muscle growth, without causing inflammation. And, thanks to the combination of olive oil, chives, garlic and lemon, it's the ultimate treat for your taste buds.

400g (14oz) firm tofu
60g (2¼oz) cashews, soaked for 2–4 hours, then drained (see page 25)
3 tbsp extra-virgin olive oil
3 tbsp fresh lemon juice
2 garlic cloves
1 tsp onion powder
Small bunch of fresh chives, finely chopped
Sea salt and black pepper
Sourdough bread, toasted, to serve (optional)

In a high-speed blender or food processor, combine the tofu, soaked cashews, olive oil, lemon juice, garlic and onion powder and season with salt and pepper. Blend until smooth, occasionally scraping down the sides.

Transfer the mixture to a bowl and fold in the finely chopped chives until evenly distributed.

Serve the spread immediately or, for the best flavour and texture, refrigerate for a few hours before serving. Enjoy on warm sourdough toast.

Notes
All spreads can be stored in an airtight container in the fridge for 5–7 days or in the freezer for up to 1 month.

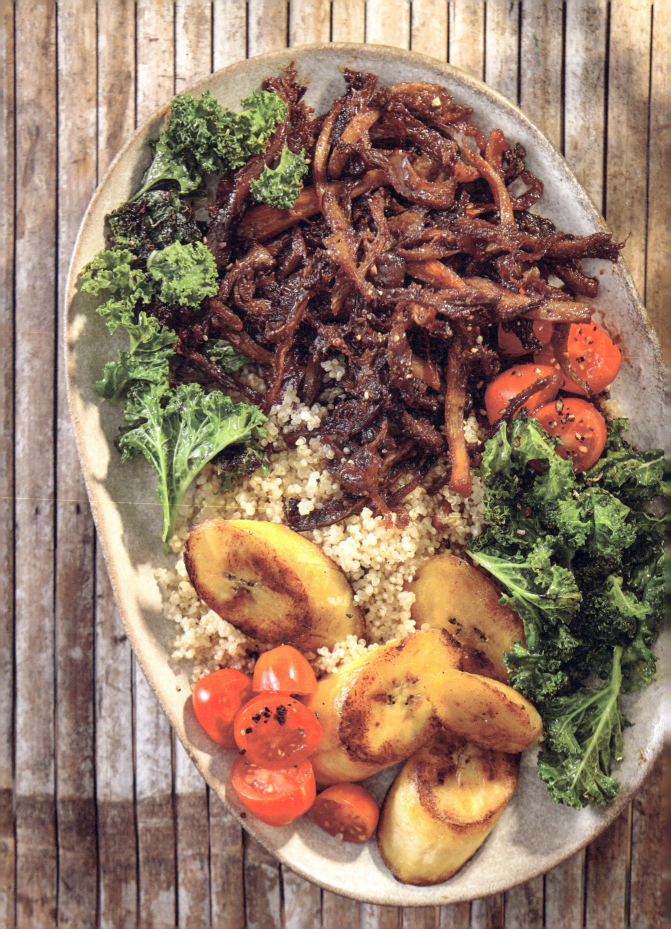

BBQ Pulled Mushrooms

Serves 2–3
Prep 5 minutes
Cook 22 minutes

Forget store-bought meat alternatives, before these processed options were available, there were mushrooms that had been doing the job naturally for centuries. With the right seasoning and technique, mushrooms turn smoky, tender and packed with umami. Roasting brings out deep, meaty flavours, while a rich, spiced glaze caramelises in the oven, creating crispy, golden edges. King oyster or oyster mushrooms work best, but any mushroom will soak up the flavour. Load these into wraps or bowls, or eat them straight from the tray. Once you try this, there's no going back.

570g (1lb 4oz) king oyster mushrooms or oyster mushrooms (button or portobello work too)
1½ tsp paprika
1½ tsp garlic powder
1½ tsp onion powder
1 tsp ground allspice
1 tsp sea salt
4 tbsp avocado oil (or any neutral oil)
120ml (4fl oz) date syrup (or 5 tbsp maple syrup)
Black pepper

Preheat the oven to Fan 200°C/220°C/425°F/Gas 7.

Using a fork or your hands, shred the mushrooms into thin strips. The more uneven and textured, the better. If you've got some help in the kitchen, now's the time to get them involved – this step takes a little patience but it's worth it.

In a large mixing bowl, combine the shredded mushrooms with the paprika, garlic powder, onion powder, allspice, salt and some pepper. Pour in the avocado oil and toss everything together until the mushrooms are evenly coated.

Transfer the mushrooms to a large baking tray and spread them out in an even layer. Roast in the preheated oven for 15 minutes, stirring halfway, until they start to shrink and take on a golden-brown colour.

Remove the tray from the oven and drizzle over the date or maple syrup. Stir well, scraping up any caramelised bits from the bottom of the tray. Spread the mushrooms out again and return to the oven for another 5–7 minutes, until the edges start to crisp up and deepen in colour.

Serve immediately – pile into wraps, stuff into sandwiches, or serve as a side. However, you use it, expect it to disappear fast.

Health Benefits

Did you know that mushrooms are neither plant nor animal? They belong to their own biological kingdom, closer to humans than plants in some ways. Unlike most plant foods, some mushrooms can provide vitamin D when exposed to sunlight and even contain small amounts of B12 – a nutrient rarely found in plant-based foods.

Raw Radiance Coleslaw

This is coleslaw but without the processed ingredients. No heavy mayo, no artificial fillers – just pure, healing food. This slaw swaps out dairy for a rich and creamy, nut-based dressing that blends with crisp cabbage and naturally sweet butternut squash. Every bite is packed with fibre, antioxidants and healthy fats, making it just as nourishing as it is delicious. A true reset for your palate.

Combine the grated squash, cabbage and spring onions in a large bowl and mix well.

In a high-speed blender or food processor, combine all the dressing ingredients and blend until smooth and creamy. Start with 100ml (3½fl oz/ scant ½ cup) coconut milk and add more, if needed, to reach the perfect consistency.

Taste and adjust the seasoning, then pour the dressing over the grated vegetables and toss everything together until well coated.

Serve immediately or set aside for 10–15 minutes to allow the flavours to meld.

½ medium butternut squash, peeled and finely grated (about 250g/9oz)

¼ head green cabbage, finely grated (about 200g/7oz)

2 spring onions (scallions), finely sliced

Creamy Cashew Dressing

150g (5½oz) cashews or Brazil nuts, soaked for 2–4 hours, then drained (see page 25)

½ spring onion (scallion)

1 tsp sea salt (adjust to taste)

100–150ml (3½–5fl oz/½ cup) coconut milk

Juice of 1 lemon

1 tbsp maple syrup

1 tbsp onion powder

1 tsp garlic powder or 1 garlic clove, minced

Black pepper

Health Benefits

This slaw is an example of what whole foods do it best. Butternut squash and cabbage provide a brilliant dose of fibre, vitamins and antioxidants to support digestion, gut health and many other systems in the body. The creamy cashew dressing delivers healthy fats and plant-based protein, making it a perfect swap for processed dressings. Soaking the nuts may also help with nutrient absorption.

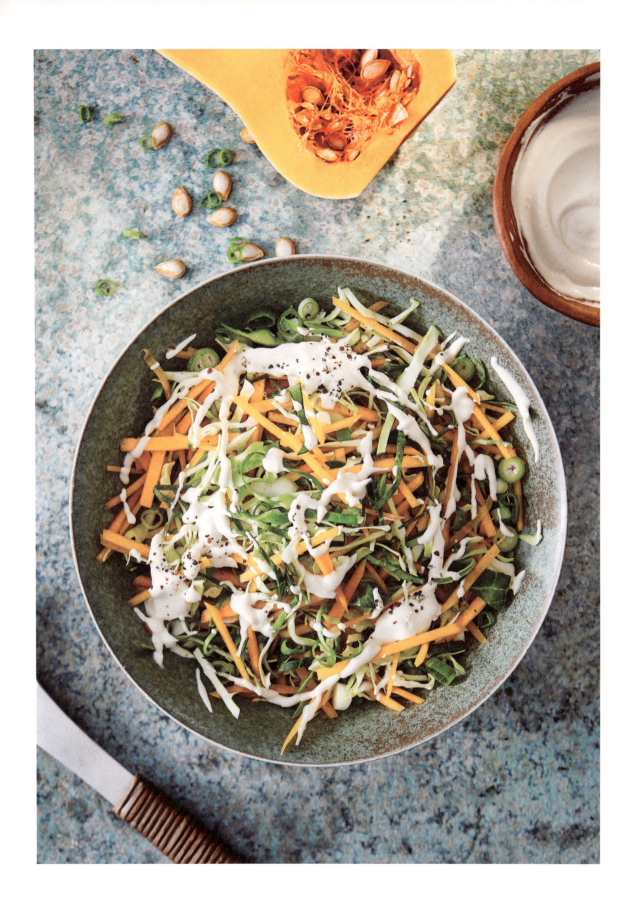

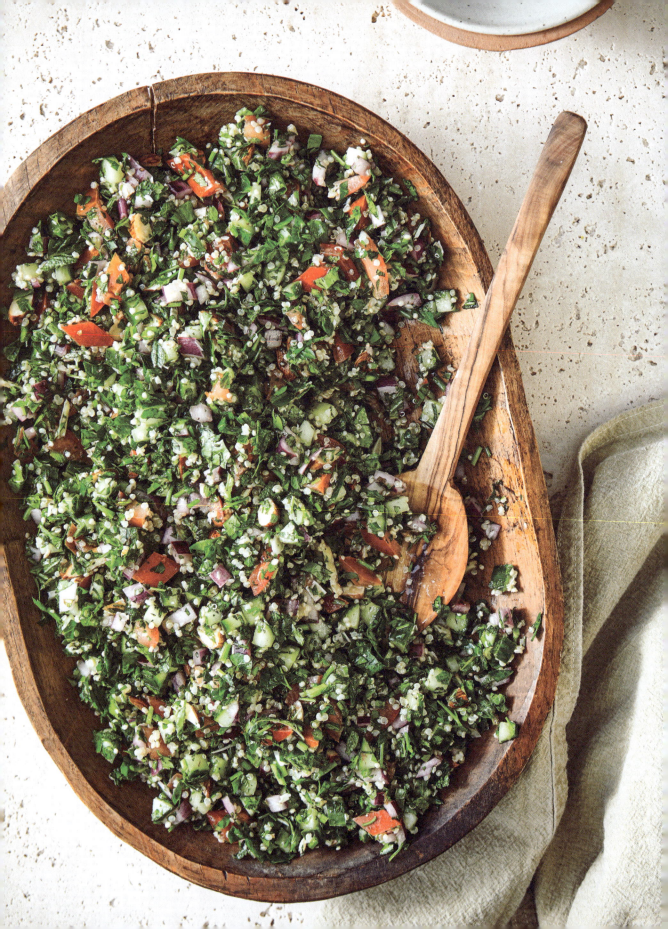

Parsley Tabbouleh

Cooking is my love language, and this dish is perfect for sharing with friends. I like to prepare a big batch and keep it in the fridge, so that I can enjoy it cold as a side or whenever I'm in the mood for something light yet satisfying. My favourite way to serve it? On romaine lettuce leaves with hummus and falafel – a simple, complete and refreshing combination.

In a large bowl, whisk together the olive oil, lemon juice, salt and pepper until well combined.

Add the cooked quinoa to the dressing and toss gently to coat it evenly. Set aside to rest for 5–10 minutes, so the quinoa can absorb the flavours.

Add the chopped parsley, tomatoes, cucumber, almonds, onion and mint to the bowl. Gently fold everything together until well combined.

Serve at room temperature or chilled. This tabbouleh pairs beautifully with hummus for a light and satisfying meal.

5 tbsp extra-virgin olive oil

3 tbsp fresh lemon juice

½ tsp sea salt

½ tsp black pepper

100g (3½oz) cooked quinoa

180g (6¼oz) fresh parsley, finely chopped

300g (10½oz) tomatoes, finely chopped

300g (10½oz) cucumber, finely chopped

50g (1¾oz) almonds, finely chopped

50g (1¾oz) red onion, finely chopped

15g (½oz) fresh mint, finely chopped

Notes

Traditionally, it is served alongside crisp salad leaves, such as romaine or iceberg, which can be used to scoop up the tabbouleh, allowing you to eat it by hand for a more authentic experience.

Turmeric Cabbage

Serves 4–6
Prep 10 minutes
Cook 20 minutes

My friend Joachim (@joachimjammeal), one of the most creative and talented chefs I know, surprised me during my visit to Guadeloupe with a dish starring a vegetable I had overlooked for most of my life – cabbage. I couldn't believe how this seemingly 'boring' vegetable could taste so incredible. The coconut oil brings out the slight sweetness of the cabbage and tomatoes, while ginger, onions, turmeric and garlic add a warm, spicy kick. In fact, it's so delicious that I ended up enjoying it on its own with just a side of avocado and rice. Serve this to your friends and they'll never look at a cabbage the same way again!

In a large skillet or wok, heat the coconut oil over a medium heat. Add the garlic, ginger, tomatoes, onion and chilli and sauté for about 5–7 minutes, stirring occasionally, until the vegetables have softened and the onion is translucent.

Add the diced cucumber and sliced red pepper, stir well and cook for another 2–3 minutes.

Stir in the finely shredded cabbage and the turmeric. Sprinkle in the salt and dried thyme, and mix everything thoroughly to combine. Cook for 5–10 minutes, stirring occasionally, until the cabbage has softened and the dish takes on a vibrant orange colour from the turmeric. The mixture should be fragrant and the flavours well combined.

Taste and adjust the seasoning, and serve warm as a side dish.

3 tbsp coconut oil
3 garlic cloves, minced
1 tbsp finely grated fresh root ginger
2 tomatoes, diced
1 brown onion, finely chopped
1 small chilli, finely chopped
1 cucumber, diced
1 red bell pepper, sliced
1 small–medium white cabbage, finely shredded
2 tbsp finely chopped fresh turmeric (or 1 tbsp ground turmeric)
1 tsp sea salt (adjust to taste)
1 tsp dried thyme
Black pepper

Health Benefits

Turmeric contains a compound called curcumin, which research has indicated may have a range of anti-inflammatory benefits, for example it may support healthy movement and functioning of your joints. Some research suggests that combining turmeric with black pepper may enhance your ability to absorb it.

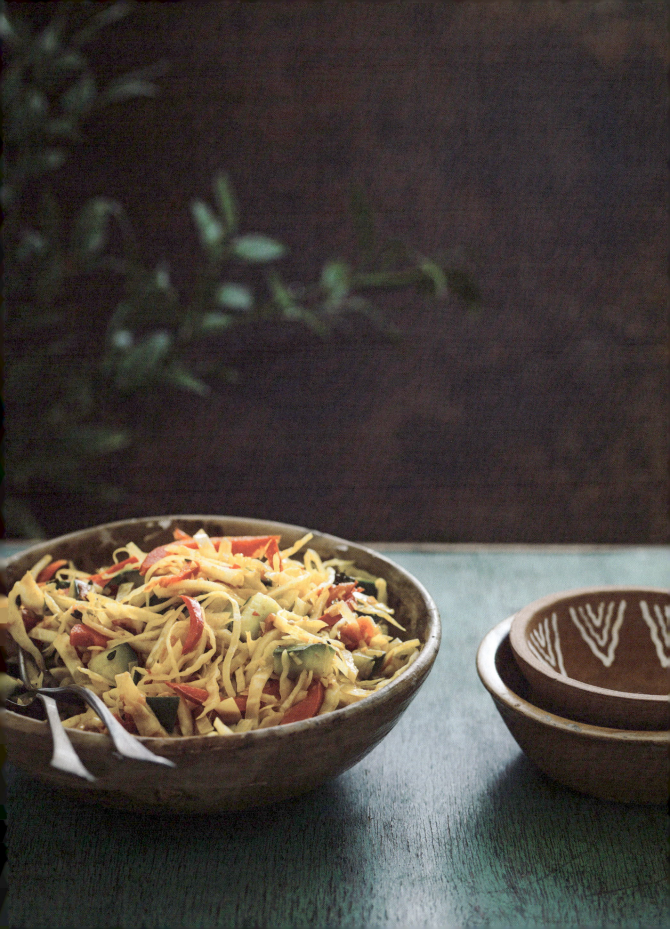

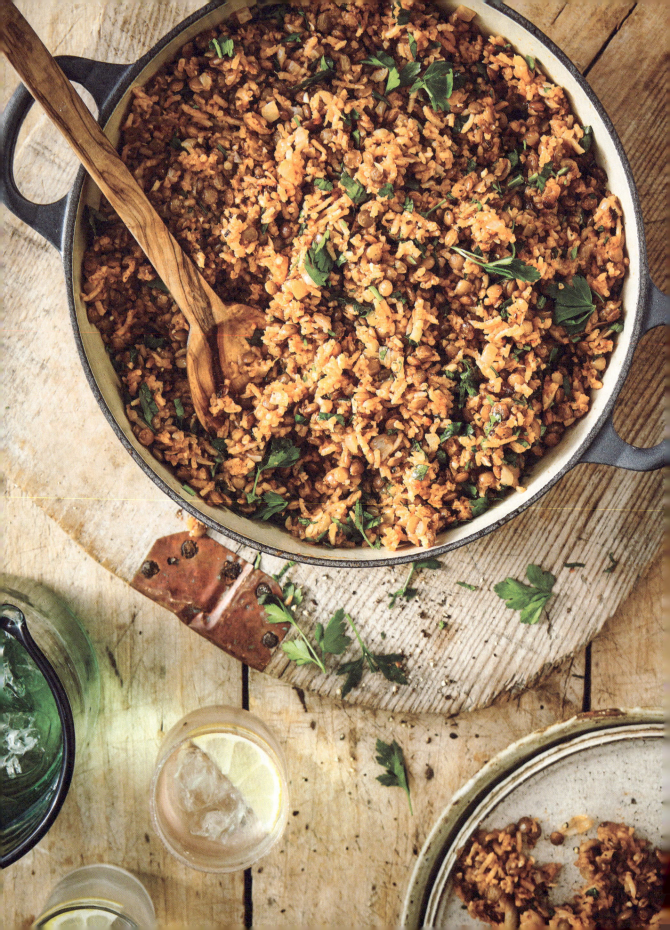

Power Packed One-Pot Lentil Rice

Serves 4–5
Prep 10 minutes
Cook 45 minutes

There's only so much we can eat in a day, so every ingredient should pull its weight. Turning a simple side like rice into something this nutrient-dense makes it a meal on its own. Packed with plant-based protein, fibre and essential minerals, this dish is comforting, filling and full of flavour. Pair it with tempeh, tofu, or a side of avocado, and you'll feel the powers.

Heat a large pot over a medium heat. Add 3–4 tablespoons of the olive oil and the onions, and sauté, stirring frequently, until the onions turn golden brown.

Lower the heat slightly and add the ginger and garlic, stirring for about 1 minute until fragrant. Be careful not to burn them.

Pour in the passata and mix well. Sprinkle in the cumin, coriander, cayenne, if using, and salt. Stir everything together and let it cook for another 2 minutes to bring out the depth of the spices.

Add the soaked lentils and rice, along with the coconut milk. Stir gently to combine, then cover with a lid and bring to a vigorous boil. Reduce the heat and simmer for 25–30 minutes, covered, until the lentils and rice are tender. If any excess moisture remains, let it cook uncovered over a low heat for another 1–2 minutes.

Remove from the heat and add the fresh parsley, lemon juice, pepper and the remaining extra-virgin olive oil. Gently fold everything together. Cover the pot and let the flavours meld for 5 minutes before serving.

5–6 tbsp extra-virgin olive oil
400g (14oz) brown onions, finely chopped
1 tbsp finely grated fresh root ginger
3 garlic cloves, finely chopped
180ml (6fl oz) passata
1 tsp ground cumin
1 tsp ground coriander
½ tsp cayenne pepper (optional)
1 tsp sea salt
200g (7oz/1 cup) brown lentils, rinsed, soaked for 4–6 hours or overnight, then drained (see page 25)
200g (7oz/1 cup) white basmati rice, rinsed, soaked for 15–30 minutes, then drained (see page 25)
475ml (17fl oz/2 cups) coconut milk
70g (2½oz) fresh parsley, finely chopped
Juice of 1 lemon or lime (adjust to taste)
Pinch of ground black pepper

Health Benefits

Lentils and rice make for the ultimate plant-based protein and fibre combo – keeping you full, energised and supporting your gut health. Lentils are naturally rich in selenium and folate, while onions bring in flavonoids that are a strong antioxidant. A drizzle of olive oil and a squeeze of lemon tie it all together, adding some healthy fats and vitamin C.

Sacred Strength Coconut Quinoa & Beans

Serves 3–4
Prep 7 minutes
Cook 18 minutes

Quinoa isn't just a grain, it's an ancient powerhouse. Considered sacred by the Incas and revered by the Mayans, quinoa was known as the 'mother of all grains', fuelling warriors and messengers on their long journeys. Unlike most grains, quinoa is a complete protein, providing all essential amino acids, making it perfect for building strength and muscle on a plant-based diet. This isn't your average side dish – with kidney beans for extra plant protein, creamy coconut milk for nourishing healthy fats, and the perfect balance of aromatic spices, this dish is satisfying, energising and built to fuel you. Whether you're aiming for muscle gains, sustained energy, or just a hearty, wholesome meal, this is the side that does it all.

2 tbsp coconut oil

3 spring onions (scallions), finely chopped, plus extra to garnish

3–4 garlic cloves, minced

200g (7oz/1 cup) quinoa, rinsed

1 × 400g (14oz) can kidney beans, drained and rinsed

1 × 400ml (14fl oz) can full-fat coconut milk

1 tsp dried thyme

1 tsp sea salt (adjust to taste)

½ tsp black pepper (adjust to taste)

¼ Scotch bonnet, finely minced, or ½ tsp cayenne pepper (optional)

Cooked plantain, to serve

Heat a large pot over a medium heat and add the coconut oil. Once melted, toss in the chopped spring onions and minced garlic, sautéing for about 2–3 minutes, until soft and fragrant.

Stir in the rinsed quinoa and kidney beans, making sure they are well coated in the aromatics. Pour in the coconut milk and 120ml (4fl oz/½ cup) water. Season with the thyme, salt, pepper and Scotch bonnet or cayenne, if using. Stir everything together to combine and bring the mixture to a gentle boil. Reduce the heat to low, cover with a lid and simmer for about 15 minutes, or until the quinoa is cooked and fluffy, absorbing the liquid.

Remove from heat and set aside, covered, for 5 minutes.

Fluff with a fork, check the seasoning and sprinkle over more spring onions. Serve warm with plantain.

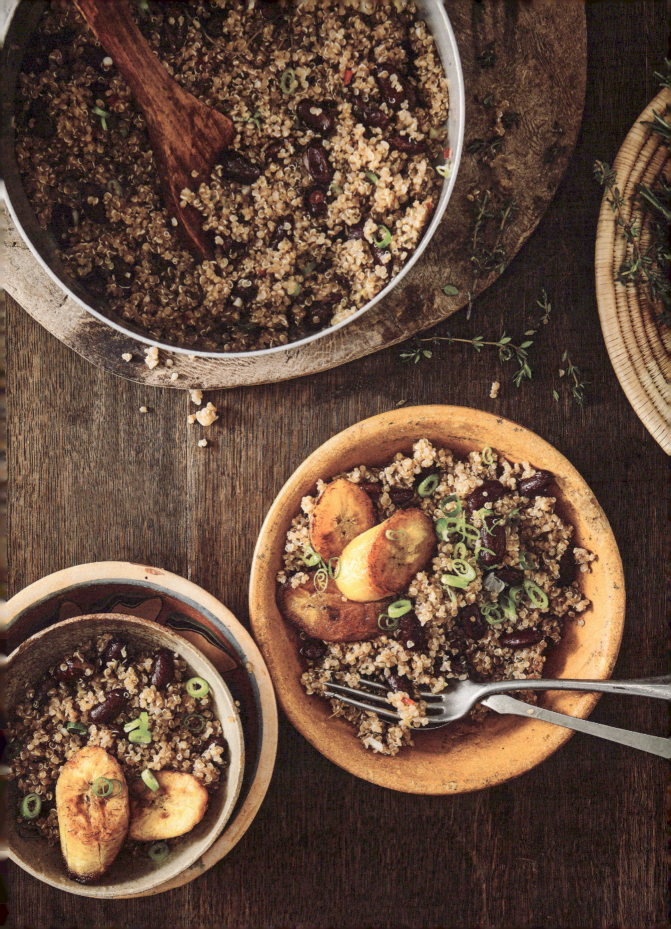

Extra-Veggie Tomato Sauce

Serves 2
Prep 10 minutes
Cook 40 minutes

A good tomato sauce is the backbone of so many meals, and once you've made it from scratch, there's no going back. This roasted tomato sauce is rich, full of depth and effortlessly sneaks in extra veggies – perfect for kids (or picky adults) who tend to avoid them. Slow-roasting the tomatoes, peppers and onions brings out a natural sweetness that makes this sauce incredibly flavourful without needing processed sugars. Toss it through your favourite pasta, spread it over pizza, or use it as a base for soups and stews. A simple, homemade staple that instantly elevates any meal.

Preheat the oven to Fan 180°C/200°C/400°F/Gas 6. Line a baking tray with parchment paper.

Place the halved tomatoes, bell pepper, onions and the nuts in a large bowl. Drizzle with the oil, then sprinkle with 1 teaspoon salt and 1 teaspoon basil. Toss until well coated.

Arrange the nuts and vegetables, cut-sides down, on the prepared baking tray and roast in the preheated oven for 30 minutes, turning halfway for even cooking. Remove from the oven and set aside to cool.

Transfer the cooled vegetables to a high-speed blender or food processor, add the medjool date and blend on high until velvety and smooth.

Pour the mixture into a large pot. Add the remaining salt and basil, as well as the oregano, onion powder and cayenne pepper, and bring to a boil. Reduce the heat and simmer for 5–10 minutes to deepen the flavours.

Serve warm as it is with your favourite pasta, or add a drizzle of coconut cream and fresh basil for extra flavour.

18 Roma tomatoes, halved
½ red bell pepper, halved and deseeded
½ brown onion, halved
½ red onion, halved
Handful of Brazil nuts (or cashews)
2 tbsp extra-virgin olive oil (or avocado oil)
1 tbsp sea salt
1 tbsp dried basil
1 medjool date, pitted
2 tsp dried oregano
2 tsp onion powder
⅛ tsp cayenne pepper

For Serving (optional)
Pasta of your choice
Coconut cream
Fresh basil leaves

Health Benefits

This sauce is packed with antioxidants, vitamins and fibre from the slow-roasted tomatoes, bell peppers and onion. Lycopene, the star compound in tomatoes, supports heart health and glowing skin. Unlike store-bought sauces that are loaded with preservatives and hidden sugars, this one keeps it pure and nourishing. A whole-food upgrade for your kitchen.

Hemp Seed Ranch Dressing

Serves 1–2
Prep 2 minutes

Some days, I like to keep it simple and let the dressing do the heavy lifting. With hemp seeds and a rich, fatty milk, this one brings both protein and healthy fats to the table. A salad is never complete without the right dressing. But, here's the twist: a good dressing shouldn't just taste great, it should elevate the nutrient profile of your salad, not weigh it down with sugars and unnecessary processed ingredients. This one does just that – it's light, nourishing and packed with intention.

In a high-speed blender or food processor, combine all the ingredients and blend on high until the mixture is smooth and creamy. Stop and scrape down the sides, as needed, to ensure everything is fully combined.

Taste and adjust the seasoning, adding more pepper, dill, or a splash more milk for your desired consistency.

Use immediately or store in an airtight container in the fridge for up to 3 days.

3 tbsp shelled hemp seeds
(or 60g/2¼oz cashews)
1 tsp onion powder
1 tsp garlic powder
1 tbsp apple cider vinegar
1 tsp maple syrup
3 tbsp oats
1 tsp dill (fresh or dried)
120ml (4fl oz/½ cup) unsweetened milk
(coconut or almond work well)
Pinch of black pepper (adjust to taste)

Health Benefits

Hemp seeds are a great source of complete plant-based protein, with just 1 tablespoon offering around 3g high-quality protein. Their mild, nutty flavour and naturally creamy, fatty texture make them a versatile, nutrient-packed base for sauces, dips, plant-based milk and hearty stews.

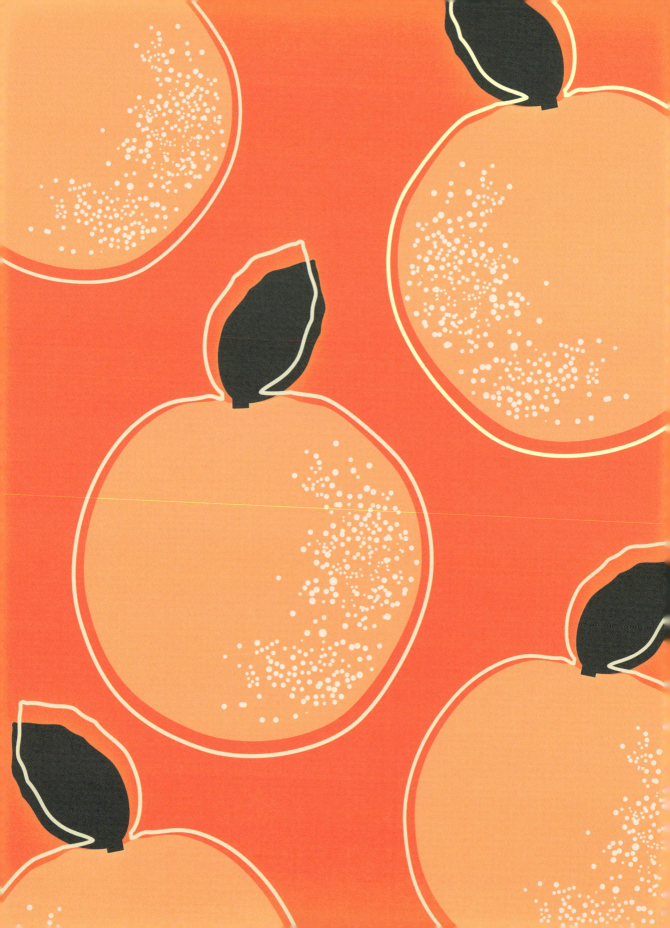

HEALING TONICS & CLEANSES

DETOX & REPLENISH

Asparagus Soup

Serves 2–4
Prep 10 minutes
Cook 40 minutes

During my twin sister's pregnancy, we explored foods known to support a healthy pregnancy, and asparagus quickly became a favourite. Rich in folate (vitamin B9), it also happened to be one of her cravings – a reminder that our bodies are constantly communicating and we just have to listen. While fresh asparagus is in season from late April to late June in the UK, it's one of those foods that retains its nutrients well when frozen, making this soup just as nourishing all year-round.

Heat the olive oil in a large pot over a medium heat. Add the onion and garlic, and sauté for 6–8 minutes, until softened and fragrant. Stir often to prevent browning, reducing the heat, if needed.

Stir in the asparagus, 700ml (24fl oz/3 cups) water and the almonds. Add the onion powder, paprika, rosemary, salt and pepper, and stir well. Increase the heat to bring the mixture to a boil, then reduce the heat, cover with a lid and simmer gently for 25–30 minutes.

Using a stick blender, purée the soup directly in the pot until smooth and creamy, or transfer to a high-speed blender or food processor.

Stir in the lemon juice, if using, to brighten the flavours. If the soup is too thick, add a little more water. If it is too thin, simmer uncovered until it reaches your desired consistency.

Ladle the soup into bowls and serve warm. For an elegant touch, you could garnish the soup with toasted almonds, a drizzle of olive oil, or a sprinkle of paprika.

2 tbsp extra-virgin olive oil, plus extra to drizzle
½ brown onion, diced
3 garlic cloves, minced
500g (1lb 2oz) asparagus, roughly chopped
75g (2¾oz) almonds
1 tsp onion powder
1 tsp paprika, plus extra to garnish
½ tsp dried rosemary
1 tsp sea salt
½ tsp black pepper
2 tbsp fresh lemon juice (optional)
Toasted flaked (slivered) almonds (optional)

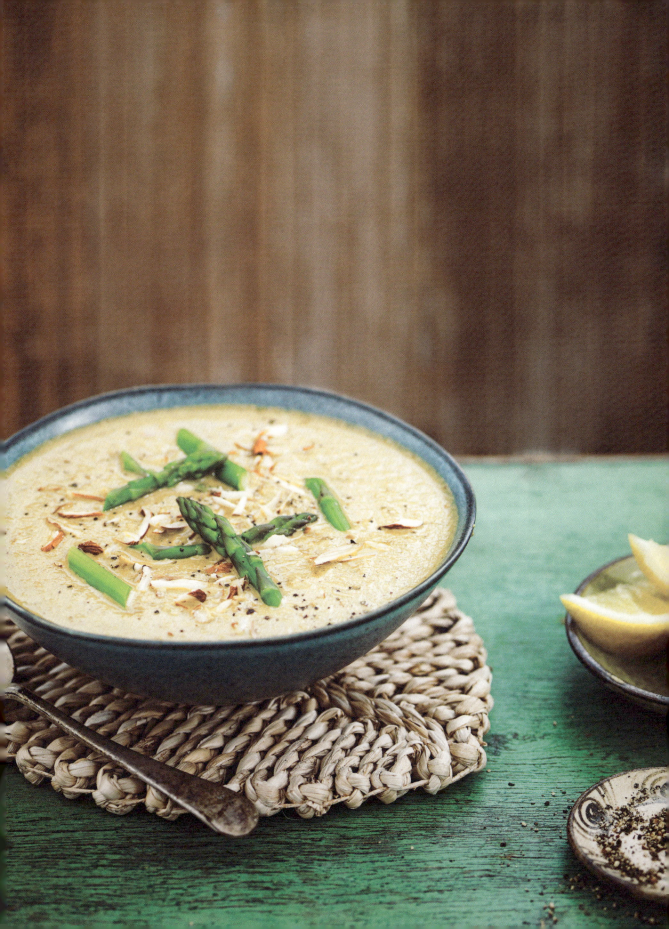

The Life Force Broth

When life feels heavy, a good broth can bring you back to centre. This isn't just any soup, it's a mineral-dense, immune-boosting elixir designed to nourish your body deeply and bring warmth to your soul. For centuries, people have turned to healing broths as a remedy for everything from fatigue to illness, and for good reason. It's like medicine, but in its most natural, soul-soothing form. Whether you sip it slowly or enjoy it as a light, warming meal, this broth is a daily ritual worth embracing. You could also blend the soup for a silky, nutrient-packed purée, or freeze it in an ice-cube tray for quick, easy servings throughout the week.

Combine all the ingredients in a large pot and pour in 2 litres (70fl oz/ 8¾ cups) water. Bring to a gentle boil, then reduce the heat and simmer for about 1 hour, allowing the flavours to deepen and the nutrients to infuse.

If you prefer a clear broth, strain it, or leave the vegetables in to enjoy it as a nourishing soup.

Season with salt and pepper, if needed, and serve warm, sipping slowly to absorb the healing benefits.

300g (10½oz) sweet potatoes, chopped
3 celery stalks, chopped
2 brown onions, sliced
30g (1oz) fresh coriander (cilantro), finely chopped
100g (3½oz) mushrooms (shiitake, portobello, or button)
2 tomatoes, chopped
6 garlic cloves, minced
Thumb-sized piece of fresh root ginger, peeled and sliced (15g/½oz)
Thumb-sized piece of fresh turmeric root, peeled and sliced (15g/½oz)
2 tsp dried thyme
½ tsp cayenne pepper (optional)
Sea salt and black pepper

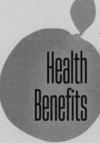

Health Benefits

This broth is packed with a wide variety of vegetables to support health and well being: carrots that are rich in beta-carotene; garlic and onions that may have antimicrobial properties; parsley and shiitake mushrooms to provide important minerals that may support your immune system. Turmeric and ginger help further with their potential anti-inflammatory properties. Every sip is a step toward healing, replenishing your body.

Pumpkin Seed Mylk

Serves 2–3
Prep 5 minutes

If you've ever felt like something's off, this milk might be exactly what you need. Soaking the pumpkin seeds is crucial – it removes enzyme inhibitors, making the nutrients more bioavailable while enhancing digestion. This milk is perfect as part of a cleanse, a morning ritual, or a post-fast drink to support a thriving, balanced body. If you're looking for an easy way to support gut health, this is a drink you'll want to add to your routine.

Drain and rinse the soaked pumpkin seeds well.

In a high-speed blender or food processor, combine all the ingredients and blend on high for 1–2 minutes until smooth. Strain the mixture through a nut milk bag or fine sieve, squeezing out all the liquid from the pulp. Otherwise, if you have a juicer with a built-in filter, run the ingredients through this.

Transfer to a glass jar and store in the fridge for up to 3 days. Shake before drinking.

50g (1¾oz) raw pumpkin seeds, soaked for 6–8 hours or overnight, then drained (see page 25)
2 medjool dates, pitted
½ tsp ground cinnamon
½ tsp ground cloves
½ tsp vanilla extract
750ml (26fl oz/3¼ cups) coconut water (or water)

Sea Moss Gel

Makes 14 doses

Sea moss is one of nature's most powerful superfoods, packed with minerals that nourish the body from the inside out. It's been used around the world for generations for its immune-boosting, gut-healing and skin-loving properties. Learning how to prepare it properly means you can unlock all of its benefits in the freshest way possible. This guide gives you two simple methods – one quick, one slow, depending on how much time you have. Whether you prefer to heat it gently the traditional way or soak it, this is the foundation for adding sea moss to your routine. Use 2 tablespoons daily in smoothies, teas, soups, or even as a natural skincare ingredient. I like to use Key limes but regular limes can also be used.

50g (1¾oz) dried sea moss
Juice of 2 limes (optional, for method 2)

Prep 5 minutes
Cook 15 minutes

Prep 4–24 hours

Method 1: Traditional Method
Rinse the sea moss thoroughly in water, using your fingers to remove any ocean particles.

Transfer the sea moss to a saucepan and cover with 500ml (18fl oz/scant 2¼ cups) fresh water. Cook over a medium heat for 10–15 minutes, until softened and a gel-like consistency. Remove from the heat and set aside to cool slightly.

Place the softened sea moss in a high-speed blender or food processor with the cooking water and blend until completely smooth. Add more water, if needed, to achieve a gel-like consistency.

Store in an airtight glass jar in the fridge for up to 3 weeks.

Method 2: Raw Method
Rinse the sea moss thoroughly in water, using your fingers to remove any ocean particles.

Place the sea moss in a glass bowl and cover with 500ml (18fl oz/scant 2¼ cups) fresh water. Add the juice of 2 limes to help balance the taste, if using. Set aside to soak for 4–24 hours, until soft and expanded.

Remove the sea moss from the water and place in a high-speed blender or food processor. Add a few tablespoons of fresh water then blend for at least 3–4 minutes, gradually adding more water, if needed, until smooth. Add more water, if needed, to achieve a gel-like consistency.

Store in a sterile, airtight glass jar in the fridge for up to 3 weeks.

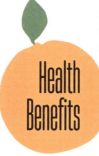

Health Benefits

Sea moss is packed with many of the minerals your body needs to thrive. It contains iodine which is important to support thyroid health, magnesium, which has an important role in energy production, and zinc which supports the health of your skin. The raw method preserves more nutrients, while the traditional method breaks it down for quicker absorption – both are great options. Pure nourishment, straight from the ocean.

146

DETOX & REPLENISH

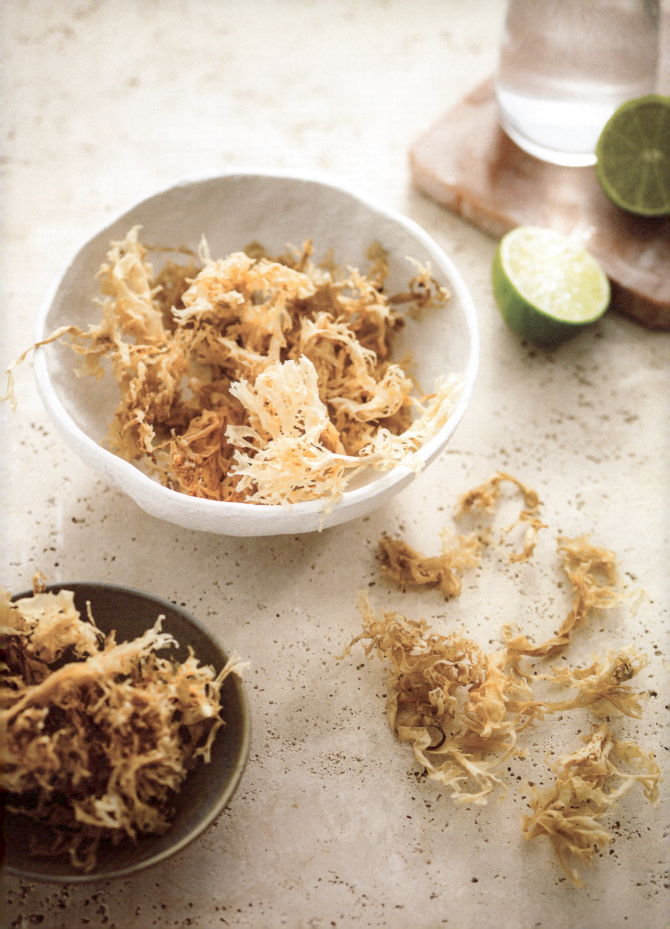

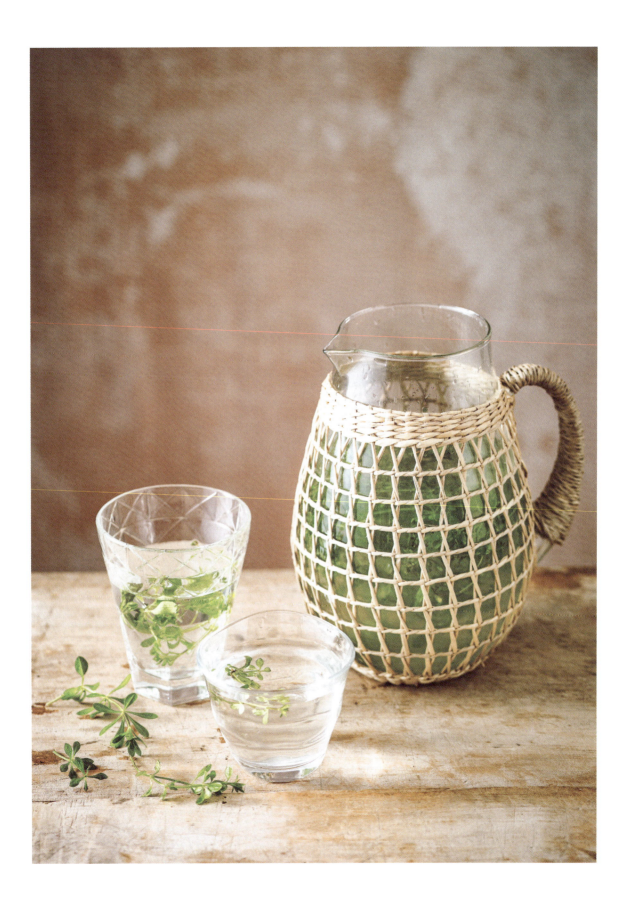

Beauty Tonic

Serves 8–10
Prep 2 hours–overnight

1 large handful of fresh young cleavers

Cleavers are in season from late winter to the end of spring. Ensure you can confidently identify cleavers before foraging – they are a sticky weed that sticks to your clothes, which makes foraging for them a fun task! According to ancient Celtic folklore, drinking cleavers water for nine weeks during spring is said to enhance your beauty so much that everyone will fall in love with you. It's perfect for clearing out any lingering sluggishness from winter. Spring cleansing herbs like cleavers are a great reminder of how living in harmony with the natural flow of the seasons and plant life can support our physical, mental and spiritual health.

Wash the cleavers thoroughly under running water to remove any dirt.

Place the cleavers in a large jug or glass jar. Pour 2 litres (3½ pints/8¼ cups) cold water over the cleavers, ensuring they are fully submerged.

Cover the jug or jar with a lid and refrigerate for at least 2 hours, or overnight, to allow the flavours and nutrients to infuse into the water.

Once infused, you can strain out the cleavers or leave them in the water, depending on your preference. Serve chilled and enjoy!

Dandelion Green Juice

Serves 1–2
Prep 5 minutes

According to ancient folklore, dandelions are known as 'elixirs of life', said to cleanse the body of negative energies. One of the most resilient plants in the world, they thrive in the harshest conditions – breaking through pavement cracks and growing in the toughest, driest soil. Considered a weed by some, millions are spent trying to eradicate them with harmful chemicals, but, in truth, there are no weeds – only flowers growing where they're not wanted. It is a beautiful plant that is nutritious, edible, medicinal and wants nothing more than to grow and greet the morning sun. We should all take a leaf out of the dandelion's book.

In a high-speed blender or food processor, combine all the ingredients, along with 100–200ml (3½–7fl oz/scant ½ cup–scant 1 cup) water. Blend until smooth. Strain the mixture using a cheesecloth or a fine-mesh sieve to separate the juice from the pulp. Otherwise, if you have a juicer with a built-in filter, run the ingredients through this, without adding water.

Transfer to a glass jar and store in the fridge for up to 3 days. Shake before drinking.

1 head of celery, chopped
2 cucumbers
2 oranges, peeled
10–15 dandelion leaves

Notes
If foraging for dandelion leaves, ensure they are correctly identified and harvested from clean, pesticide-free areas. Use the entire leaf, including the stalk. Adjust the amount of water, if blending, depending on your preferred consistency.

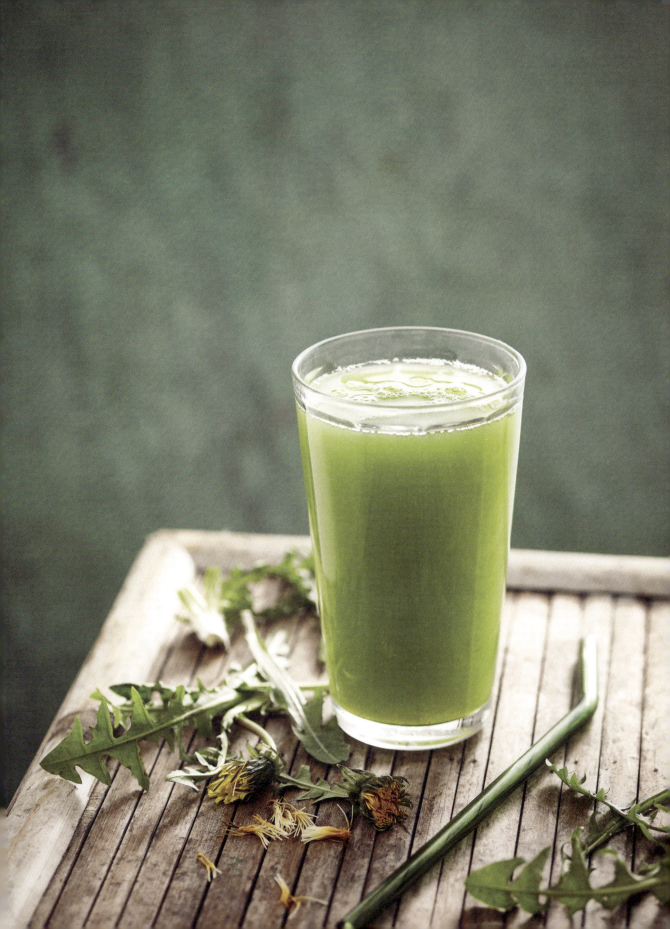

Wake Up Call

My grandpa introduced me to this one. Back in the Nigerian army, when coffee wasn't always available, they had their own way of firing up the body before long days – they called them 'Firebreath Shots'. A quick hit of cayenne pepper and lime juice, straight to the system. No caffeine, no crash – just pure, clean fire. Take this shot first thing in the morning or before a workout and feel the buzz – warmth spreading through your body, blood flowing, energy rising. No coffee needed.

Juice of 1 lime (enough to fill a shot glass)
¼ tsp cayenne pepper

Combine the lime juice and cayenne pepper in a shot glass. Mix well.

Take it as a shot – quick, fiery and straight to the system.

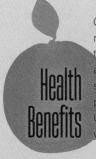

Health Benefits

Cayenne pepper contains a compound called capsaicin, responsible for its spicy flavour. Some research indicates that it may also have a positive impact on blood pressure and it is known for its ability to stimulate blood flow, support heart health and fire up metabolism. The lime juice provides a natural hit of vitamin C and other antioxidants. Unlike caffeine, which spikes and crashes, this shot gives you the wake up call without the jitters.

Defender Tonic

This should be your first line of defence when you feel something coming on. This isn't just a warm drink, it's nature's way of fighting back. Ginger, with its fiery kick, has been used for centuries to boost immunity, fight inflammation and improve circulation. This is the drink to break your fast, fight off colds before they start, or just keep your system strong – a simple but powerful ritual for daily resilience.

Thumb-sized piece of fresh root ginger, peeled and grated
Juice of 1 lime

Place the ginger and 500ml (18fl oz/scant 2¼ cups) water in a small saucepan and bring to a boil. Reduce the heat and simmer for 10–15 minutes, to extract the ginger's benefits fully.

Strain the liquid into a cup and set aside to cool slightly.

Squeeze in the fresh lime juice and stir.

Drink warm on an empty stomach and let the body do the rest.

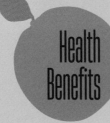

Health Benefits

Ginger has natural antimicrobial properties; its fiery taste can do wonders for sore throats and colds. The lime in this recipe is a great source of vitamin C, a key nutrient for supporting our immune system as well as our skin health.

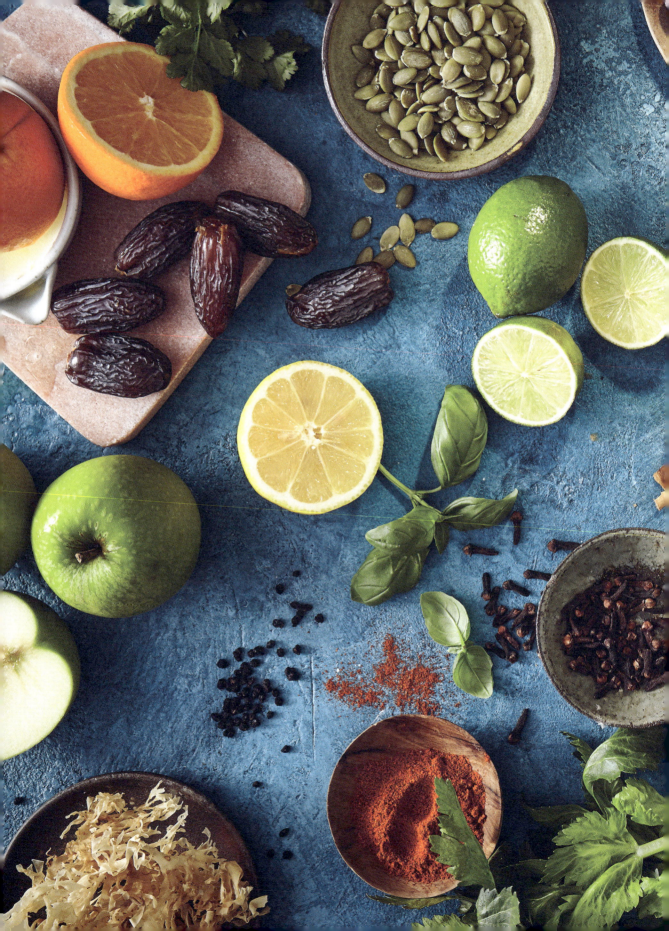

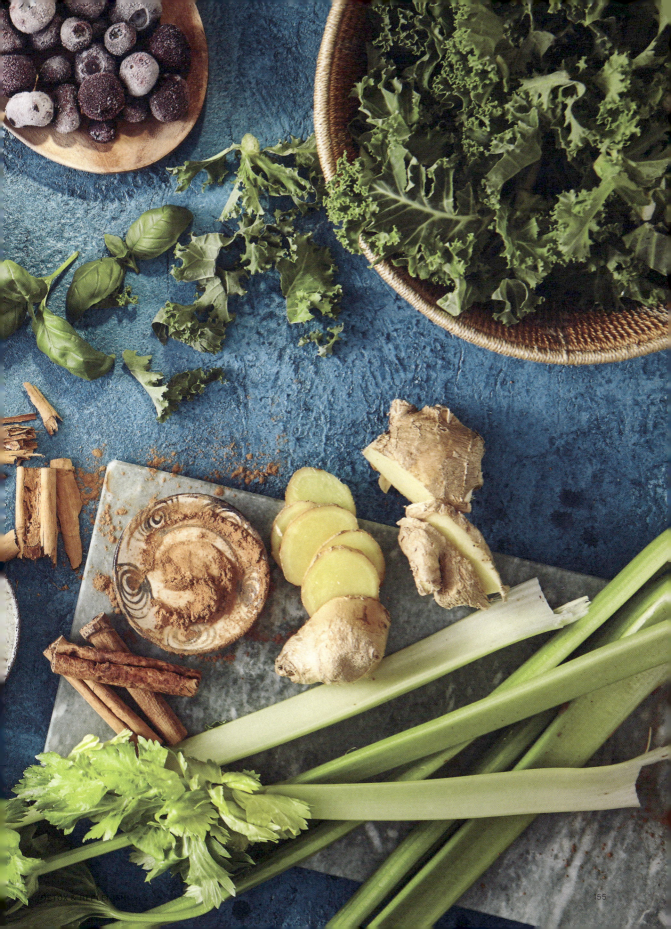

Celery Tonic

Serves 1–2
Prep 5 minutes

Some things in life work so well, you wonder why you didn't start sooner. Celery juice is one of them. For me, it started as a simple experiment – one glass first thing in the morning, before anything else. No expectations, just curiosity. Within days, my digestion felt lighter, my skin looked clearer and my energy was different – a clean, steady buzz that lasted all day. Celery might seem basic, but don't be fooled. Beneath its crisp, refreshing taste, the juice acts like a deep, internal cleanse, clearing out what doesn't belong and flooding your body with hydration, minerals and vitality. The first sip might surprise you, but soon, you'll crave it.

1 large head of celery (organic if possible), roughly chopped
Squeeze of fresh lemon juice (optional)

In a high-speed blender or food processor, add the celery with 250–500ml (9–18fl oz/1–2 cups) water. Blend until smooth. Strain through a nut milk bag or fine-mesh sieve. Otherwise, if you have a juicer with a built-in filter, pass the celery through this, without adding water.

Pour the celery juice into a glass and drink immediately. If you're still adjusting to the taste, you can add a squeeze of lemon juice to balance the flavour.

Heavy Metal Combat Smoothie

Serves 1
Prep 5 minutes

Toxic heavy metals are everywhere – in the foods we eat (pesticides), cookware, aluminium cans and foil, and even in batteries. In today's world, it's nearly impossible to avoid them entirely, even with a strict organic and unprocessed diet. Thankfully, foods like wild blueberries, coriander and sea moss can support the body's natural detoxification processes and help combat the effects of heavy metals. This smoothie combines these powerful ingredients to nourish your body and aid in gentle cleansing.

In a high-speed blender or food processor, combine all the ingredients. Blend on high until smooth.

Gradually add the coconut water or the same amount of water, 2 tablespoons at a time, blending between additions, until it reaches your desired consistency.

Pour the smoothie into a glass and serve immediately. Enjoy chilled.

2 ripe bananas

250g (9oz) frozen or fresh wild blueberries

40g (1½oz) fresh coriander (cilantro)

2 tbsp sea moss gel (see page 146)

Juice of 2 oranges (about 150ml/ 5fl oz/⅔ cup)

120–240ml (4–9fl oz/½–1 cup) coconut water (optional)

Notes

If wild blueberries aren't available, foraged or store-bought blackberries make a great substitute. If you prefer a sweeter flavour, add an extra banana or another freshly squeezed orange to enhance the natural sweetness.

Homemade Cough Syrup

Makes 15 doses
Prep 5 minutes
Cook 1 hour

Does medicine really grow on trees? Hippocrates famously said, 'Let food be thy medicine and medicine be thy food.' Elderberries are a perfect reminder of this wisdom. Only a few generations ago, the earth was our pharmacy, with the land providing remedies for countless ailments. Your grandparents can probably still put together a basic essential healing kit using a few local herbs. I always keep a jar of elderberry syrup in my fridge – it lasts for months and is my go-to whenever I feel under the weather. At the first sign of a scratchy throat or the onset of a cold, I take 1–2 tablespoons as a preventative - proof that nature still holds the answers, if we know where to look.

110g (3¾oz) dried elderberries
15g (½oz) fresh root ginger, peeled and grated
10g (¼oz) whole cloves
1 stick cinnamon
½ tsp cayenne pepper
120ml (4fl oz) raw honey, agave syrup, or maple syrup

Bring 850ml (29fl oz/3½ cups) water to a boil in a saucepan over a high heat.

Add the elderberries, ginger, cloves, cinnamon and cayenne pepper, reduce the heat to low-medium and simmer gently for 45–60 minutes, or until the liquid has reduced by half. Remove the saucepan from the heat and set aside to cool for 15–20 minutes.

Strain the liquid through a fine-mesh sieve or cheesecloth into a clean bowl, pressing the solids to extract as much liquid as possible. Stir the honey, agave or date syrup into the liquid until fully dissolved.

Pour the syrup into a glass jar and store in the fridge for up to 2 months.

Take 1–2 tablespoons daily, preferably with herbal tea in the morning, to support your immune system.

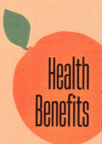

Health Benefits

Elderberries are a great source of antioxidants and vitamin C. These nutrients have an important role in supporting the healthy functioning of our immune system. Always ensure elderberries are cooked, as raw elderberries can be toxic. Consume this daily leading up to the winter to boost your immune system.

Green Living Water

Once I started getting more greens into my diet, my skin changed – glowing, soft, and more vibrant than ever. A few weeks of consistently eating leafy greens with dinner or juicing them in the mornings, and I could literally see and feel the difference. But it wasn't just about the glow – greens helped reset my taste buds, making me crave simple, natural foods again. Leafy greens have a way of resetting the body, and this juice makes it effortless to get them in first thing in the morning.

In a high-speed blender or food processor, combine all the ingredients with 100–200ml (3½–7fl oz/scant ½–1 cup) of the coconut water. Blend on high until smooth. Strain the mixture using a cheesecloth or fine-mesh sieve to separate the juice from the pulp. Otherwise, if you have a juice with a built-in filter, run the kale, romaine lettuce, coriander, basil and apples through the juicer.

Pour the juice into a jug and stir in a small amount of coconut water to combine. Add more, if needed, to reach your preferred taste and consistency.

Pour the green living water into a glass and enjoy immediately.

2 large handfuls kale (approx. 40g/1½oz), stalks removed

2 large handfuls romaine lettuce (approx. 50g/1¾oz)

10g (¼oz) fresh coriander (cilantro) (about ¼ cup, loosely packed)

10g (¼oz) fresh basil (about ¼ cup, loosely packed)

2 green apples, chopped

250ml (9fl oz/generous 1 cup) coconut water (adjust as needed)

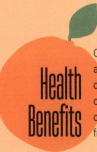

Health Benefits

Chlorophyll. the green pigment in plants, also has antioxidant properties that may protect against free radical damage. Found in leafy greens, like kale, spinach or coriander (cilantro), and sea vegetables, like sea moss, it's a direct shot of plant-powered goodness. Simple and straight from the earth.

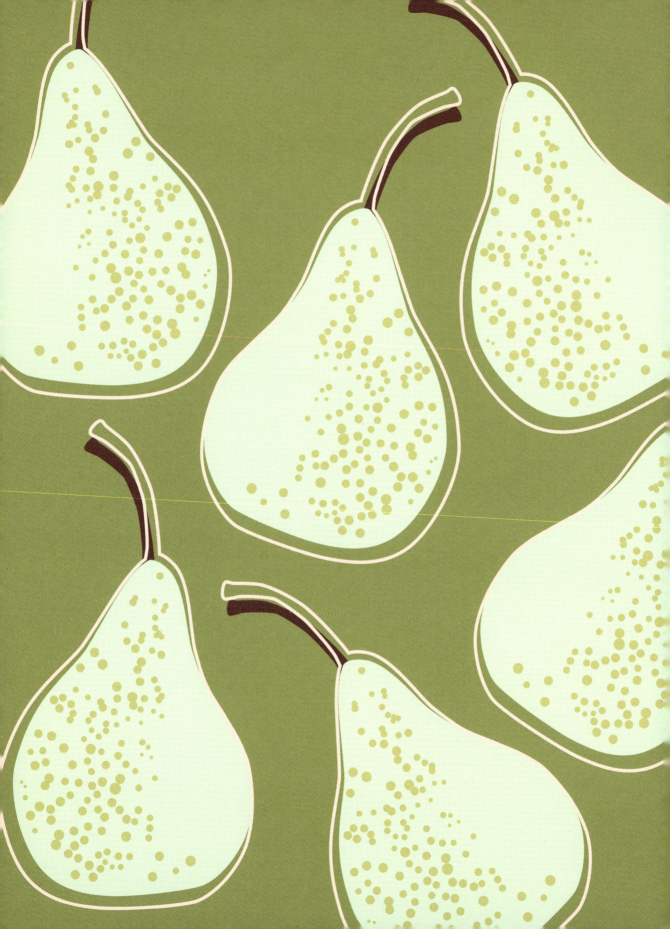

TREATS WITH BENEFITS

SWEET

Gluten–Free Sweet Potato Brownies

Makes 9
Prep 20 minutes
Cook 1 hour

Sweet potatoes in brownies? It might sound unusual, but hear me out. With a sweet tooth like mine, one of my favourite weekend activities is transforming guilty pleasures into guilt-free delights. I've experimented with countless brownie recipes – adding chickpeas, carrot, apple sauce, you name it. But nothing quite compares to the fudgy texture and boost you get from sweet potatoes. Their creamy consistency makes them a perfect substitute for butter or eggs, and their natural sugars add a subtle sweetness. Proof that limitations often spark the best creativity!

Preheat the oven to Fan 160°C/180°C/350°F/Gas 6. Line a 20cm (8in) square baking tin with parchment paper.

Steam or boil the sweet potato chunks for about 10–15 minutes, until fork-tender. Drain and leave to cool slightly.

Place the cooked sweet potatoes and medjool dates in a food processor and blend until a smooth, sticky purée.

Combine the ground almonds, ground oats, melted coconut oil, cacao powder, cinnamon, cloves, maple syrup and a pinch of sea salt in a large mixing bowl. Stir in the sweet potato and date purée until it forms a thick batter.

Spread the brownie batter evenly into the prepared tin, smoothing out the surface with a spatula. Bake in the preheated oven for 45 minutes, or until a knife inserted in the middle comes out clean. Remove from the oven and leave the brownies to cool in the tin for about 10 minutes.

Meanwhile, to make the icing, whisk together the ingredients in a small bowl, until smooth and glossy. You can melt this down in a small pan over a low heat to help get a smooth texture, if preferred. Leave at room temperature or place in the fridge briefly to thicken slightly.

Once the brownies are completely cool, spread the icing evenly over the top. Sprinkle over the crushed walnuts, slice into squares and enjoy!

Store in an airtight container for up to 5 days.

500g (1lb 2oz) sweet potato, peeled and cut into chunks
10 medjool dates, pitted
100g (3½oz/generous ¾ cup) ground almonds
100g (3½oz/generous 1 cup) oats, ground
2 tbsp coconut oil, melted
6 tbsp raw cacao powder
1 tsp ground cinnamon
½ tsp ground cloves
7 tbsp pure maple syrup
Pinch of sea salt
2 handfuls walnuts, crushed, to decorate

Icing
2 tbsp coconut oil, melted
3 tbsp maple syrup
2 tbsp raw cacao powder
2 tbsp tahini

Health Benefits

Sweet potatoes take the place of traditional refined flour here, making these brownies naturally rich in fibre, vitamins and minerals. They bring a subtle sweetness and a soft, fudgy texture, while also providing complex carbohydrates to sustain energy levels. Cacao adds polyphenols and antioxidants, while ground almonds and oats bring in healthy fats and fibre to keep you satisfied.

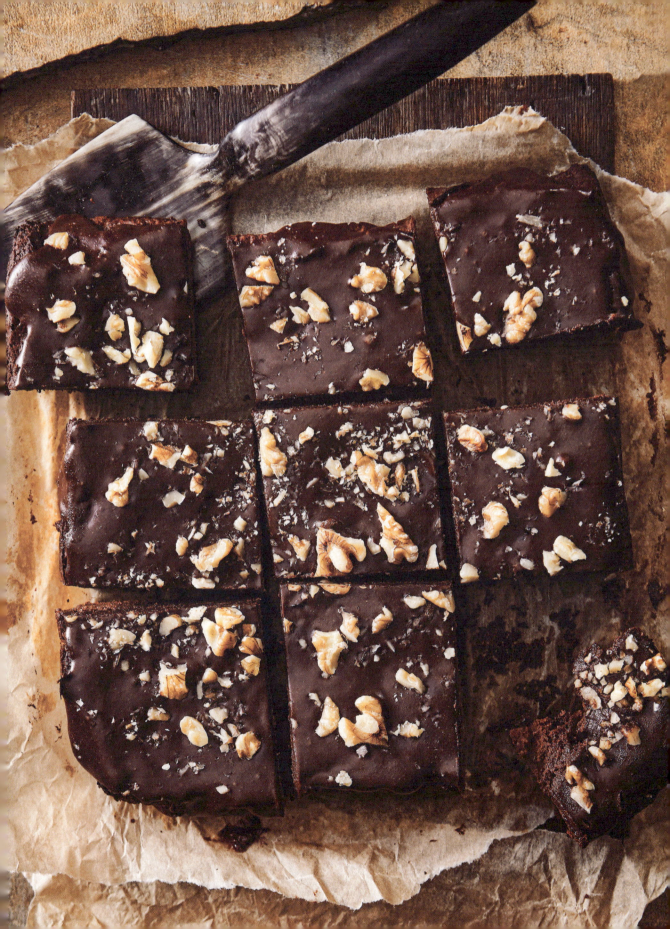

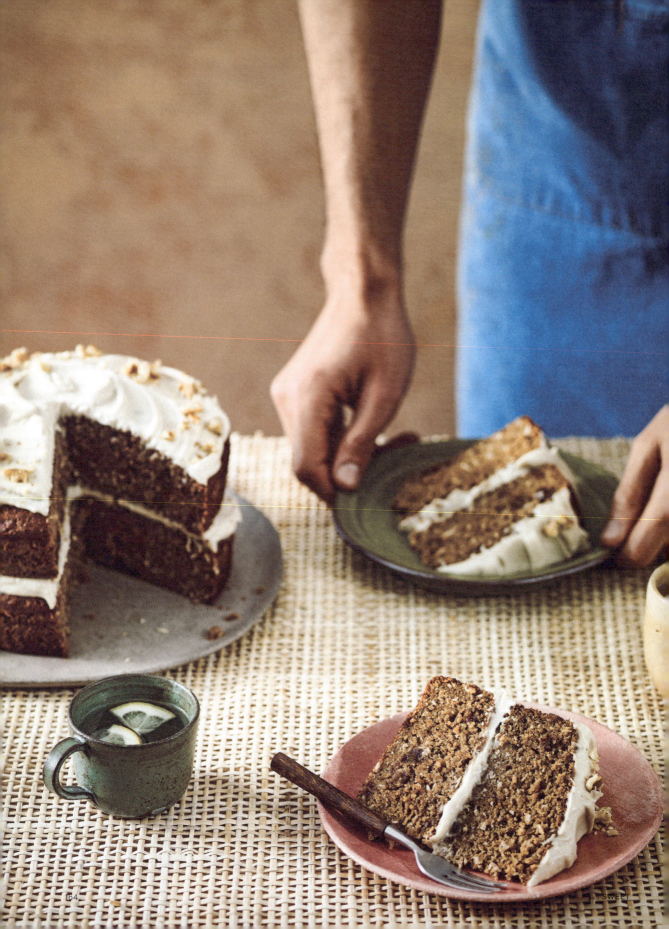

My Sister's Carrot Cake

Serves 6–8
Prep 15 minutes
Cook 40 minutes

My sister has always had that effortless glow – healthy, vibrant and full of life. She's a mum to a one-year-old, juggling everything while making it look easy. This cake is hers. A naturally sweet, spiced carrot cake, packed with real ingredients and topped with the creamiest cashew frosting. No refined sugar, no fillers – just food that feels indulgent but actually nourishes. A cake that's good enough to eat straight from the fridge (if it makes it that far). Bake this for your people and they'll remember you for it – because some cakes aren't just dessert, they're an experience.

Preheat the oven to Fan 160°C/180°C/350°F/Gas 6. Grease two 23cm (9in) cake tins with coconut oil and set aside.

In a large mixing bowl, combine the flour, baking powder, bicarbonate of soda, ground almonds, desiccated coconut, ground cloves, ginger, cinnamon and date sugar, and mix until evenly combined.

Add the grated carrots and chopped dates, then pour in the milk and melted coconut oil. Stir everything together to a well-mixed batter.

Divide evenly between the two prepared cake tins and level the surfaces. Bake for 30–40 minutes, or until a knife inserted into the centre comes out clean. If they need more time, bake for a few more minutes and check again.

Remove the cakes from the oven and leave to cool completely in their tins – this helps them firm up and prevents crumbling.

Meanwhile, prepare the frosting. Drain and rinse the soaked cashews, then add them to a high-speed blender or food processor with the maple syrup, milk and vanilla extract, if using. Blend until completely smooth. If the frosting feels too thick, add a splash more milk, but keep it thick enough to hold well on the cake.

Once the cakes are fully cooled, carefully remove them from the tins. Spread half the frosting over the first cake, then place the second cake on top. Cover with the remaining frosting. Decorate with crushed pistachios, or any toppings of your choice, such as fresh strawberries.

Slice, serve and enjoy.

100g (3½oz) coconut oil, melted, plus extra for greasing

400g (14oz/3 cups) white spelt flour (or buckwheat flour, for a gluten-free alternative)

2 tsp baking powder

1 tsp bicarbonate of soda (baking soda)

200g (7oz/scant 1¾ cups) ground almonds

75g (2¾oz/scant 1 cup) desiccated (dried shredded) coconut

½ tsp ground cloves

½ tsp ground ginger

1 tsp ground cinnamon

400g (14oz) date sugar (or coconut sugar)

3 carrots, finely grated

100g (3½oz) medjool dates, pitted and finely chopped

625ml (21½fl oz/2 ⅔ cups) unsweetened milk of choice (coconut or almond work well)

Frosting

250g (9oz) cashews, soaked for 4–6 hours, then drained (see page 25)

6–8 tbsp maple syrup

2 tbsp unsweetened milk of choice (coconut or almond work well)

1 tsp vanilla extract (optional)

Decoration

Crushed pistachos (optional)

Fresh strawberries (optional)

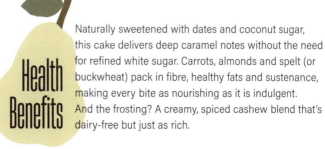

Health Benefits

Naturally sweetened with dates and coconut sugar, this cake delivers deep caramel notes without the need for refined white sugar. Carrots, almonds and spelt (or buckwheat) pack in fibre, healthy fats and sustenance, making every bite as nourishing as it is indulgent. And the frosting? A creamy, spiced cashew blend that's dairy-free but just as rich.

Apple Pie in a Glass

The pure sweetness of fresh apple juice has long been known to lift the spirit, offering comfort, warmth and a sense of ease. This smoothie is all about indulgence without compromise – a healthy way to satisfy sweet cravings while fuelling your body with nourishing ingredients. It gives you that cozy, spiced apple pie flavour, but without the processed ingredients that usually come with it. A blend of warming cinnamon, fresh apples and creamy banana, it's the kind of treat that makes you feel both comforted and energised. Next time the sweet cravings hit, skip the processed desserts and make this instead. Your body – and your taste buds – will thank you.

2 red apples, cut into small chunks
1 frozen banana
1 tsp ground cinnamon
½ tsp ground cloves
Pinch of ground nutmeg
1 tbsp maple syrup or 1 medjool date, pitted (optional)

In a high-speed blender or food processor, combine all the ingredients with 225ml (8fl oz/scant 1 cup) water and blend until smooth. If it's too thick, add a splash more water. If you like it sweeter, add an extra date or a drizzle more maple syrup.

Pour into a glass and enjoy straight away.

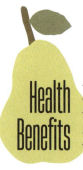

Health Benefits

Apples don't just taste good, they come packed with antioxidants, fibre and natural sugars that provide a steady source of energy without the crash.

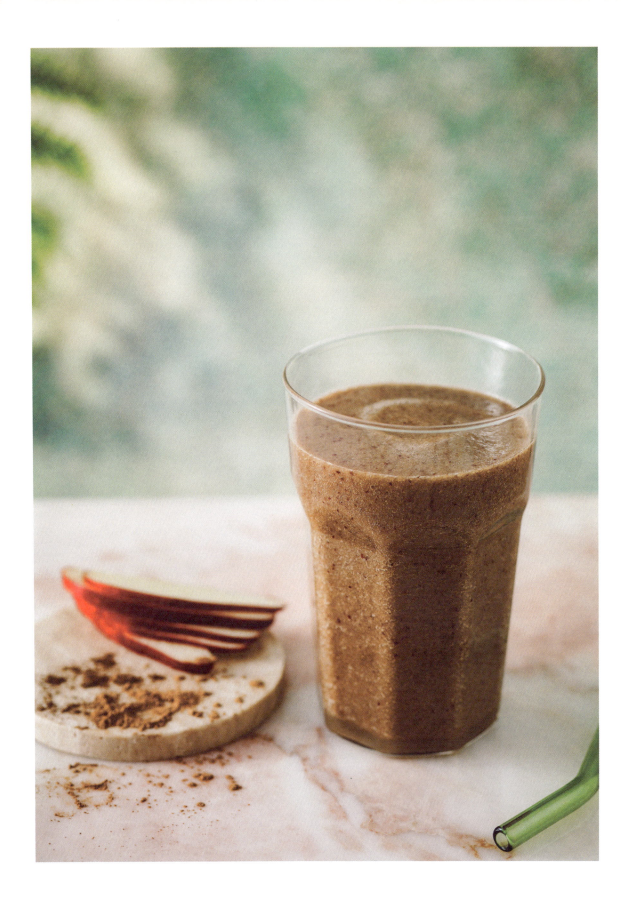

Raw Cheesecake

Creating dishes using foods in their natural, raw state requires a bit of creative thinking. What some may see as a limitation, others see as an opportunity to innovate. Curiosity led me to experiment with only raw, natural foods. The results? A newfound love and appreciation for food, a glow from within that shone through my skin and – my favourite takeaway – this raw cheesecake recipe that I developed during my cleanse.

For the crust, in a food processor, combine the almonds, walnuts, oats, carrots, dates, cinnamon and cloves. Blend until the mixture sticks together but remains slightly coarse.

Press the mixture into the base of a 23cm (9in) springform tin to make an even crust.

In a high-speed blender or food processor, combine the soaked cashews, coconut milk, honey, coconut oil and lime juice. Blend until smooth and creamy. Pour the filling over the crust and level the surface.

If making the icing, combine the mango, honey and coconut oil in a high-speed blender. Blend until smooth, then drizzle over the filling.

Freeze the cheesecake for 3–4 hours or overnight.

Defrost at room temperature for 15–30 minutes before slicing. Serve with fresh strawberries, if desired.

Crust

150g (5½oz) almonds
120g (4¼oz) walnuts
40g (1½oz/scant ½ cup) rolled oats
60g (2¼oz) carrots, grated
75g (2¾oz) medjool dates, pitted
1 tsp ground cinnamon
¼ tsp ground cloves

Filling

300g (10½oz) cashews, soaked for 4–6 hours, then drained (see page 25)
320ml (11fl oz/1 ⅓ cups) full-fat coconut milk
5 tbsp raw honey (or maple or agave syrup)
2 tbsp coconut oil, melted
Juice of 2 limes

Icing (optional)

300g (10½oz) mango (fresh or frozen)
1 tbsp raw honey (or maple or agave syrup)
20g (¾oz) coconut oil, melted
Fresh strawberries, to decorate

Note

This raw cake can be stored in the freezer for up to 3 months. For best results, freeze the cake whole, then let it defrost just once before slicing into individual portions. Once sliced, return the slices to the freezer in an airtight container. This way, you can defrost one slice at a time, as needed, avoiding multiple defrost cycles, which can affect the texture and quality.

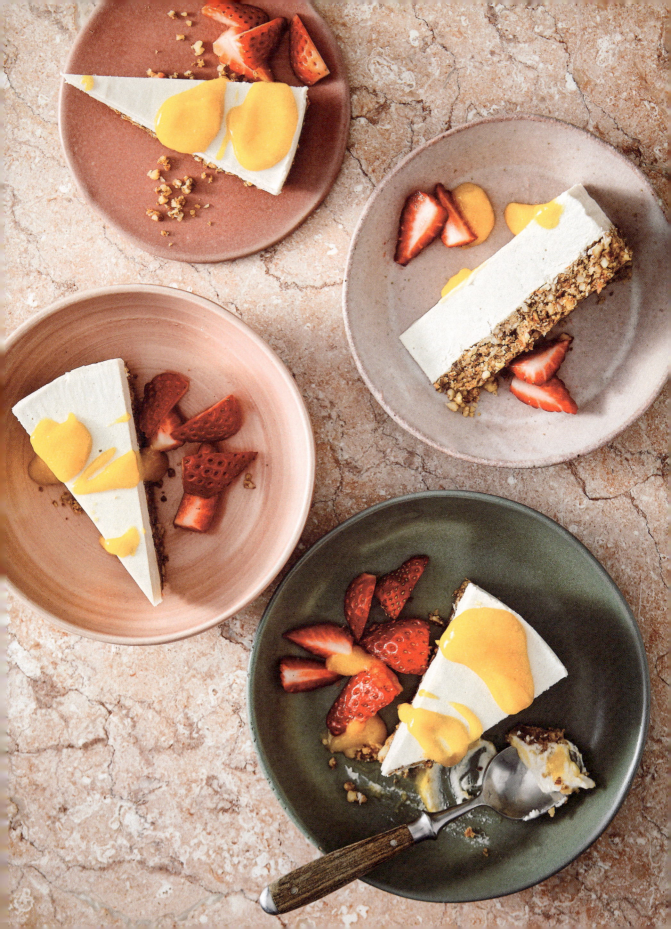

Cinnamon Baked Pears

Roasted walnuts, cinnamon-baked pears and warm maple syrup – it's like a cozy autumn hug. The nutty, warm sweetness filling the kitchen is a favourite with my younger siblings and parents alike.

Preheat the oven to Fan 160°C/180°C/350°F/Gas 6.

Cut the pears in half lengthwise and remove the seeds using a spoon.

Place the pear halves in a baking dish. Drizzle them with maple syrup and sprinkle generously with cinnamon and ground cloves. Toss gently to ensure they are evenly coated.

Fill the hollow of each pear half with crushed walnuts, pressing lightly to keep them in place. Bake the pears in the preheated oven for 20–30 minutes, or until they are soft and tender when pierced with a fork.

Serve warm, sprinkled with more crushed walnuts for added texture and flavour.

4 pears
2 tbsp maple syrup
2 tsp ground cinnamon
½ tsp ground cloves
30g (1oz) walnuts, crushed,
  plus extra to garnish

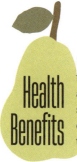

Health Benefits

Pears are one of my favourite morning foods. They are fibre rich, which helps add bulk to bowel movements and stimulates gut movement, making it easier to empty the bowels and start the day feeling lighter.

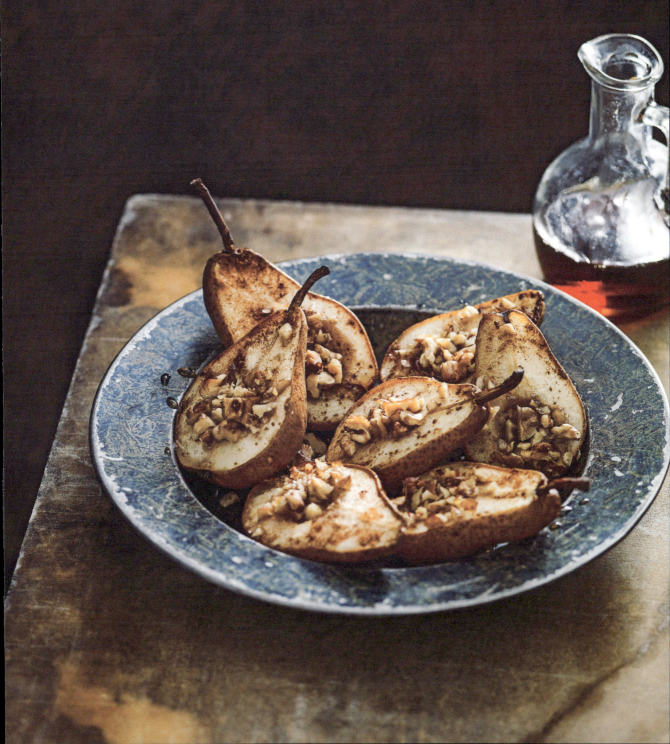

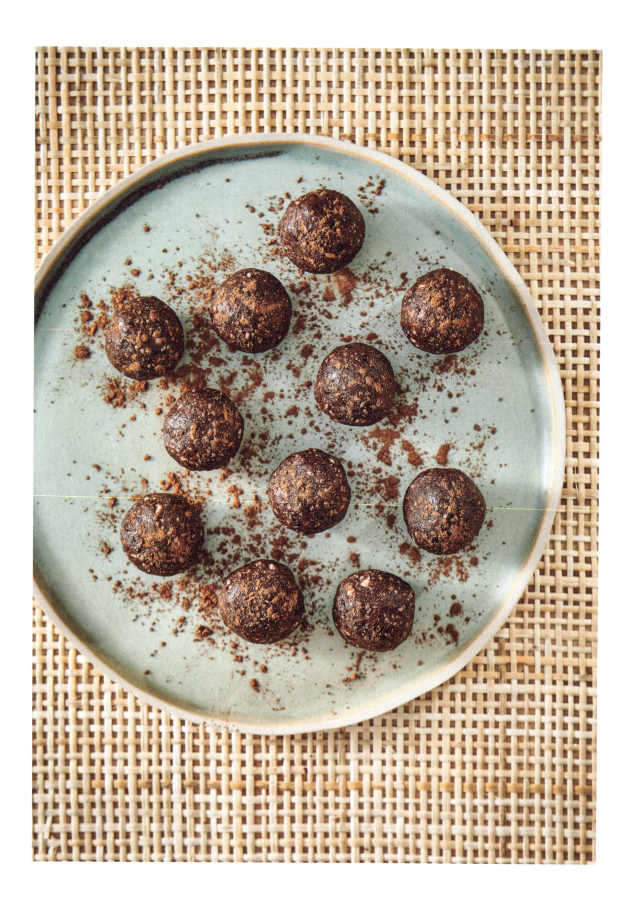

Raw Power Bites

Some snacks just make sense – quick to make, packed with goodness and naturally satisfying. These cacao power bites are exactly that. With a deep cacao flavour, natural sweetness from dates and a creamy hint of tahini, it all comes together in minutes with no baking needed. Just simple, real ingredients that keep you fuelled without the crash. Keep a batch in the fridge and you'll always have something to grab when you need an energy boost - pre-workout, mid-afternoon, or straight from the fridge when the cravings hit.

100g (3½oz) almonds
200g (7oz) medjool dates, pitted
2 tbsp raw cacao powder, plus optional extra for sprinkling
1 tbsp coconut oil
1 tbsp tahini

Put the almonds in a food processor and pulse a few times until broken down into a coarse crumb.

Add the dates, cacao powder, coconut oil and tahini, then blend until everything starts to come together into a sticky dough. If needed, stop to scrape down the sides and blend again. Check if it's ready by pressing a small amount between your fingers – it should hold its shape easily.

Roll the mixture into small balls, roughly half the size of a golf ball. Sprinkle with more cacao before serving, if desired.

Store in an airtight container in the fridge for up to 2 weeks, or in the freezer for up to 3 months.

Health Benefits

Nature's energy boost, dates provide natural sugars but, unlike refined sugar, they come with fibre, vitamins and minerals and release energy more slowly. Raw cacao is more than just chocolate – it's packed with magnesium, iron and antioxidants. Nutrient-dense fats in the almonds, tahini and coconut oil keep these bites satisfying and help support slow release, longer-lasting energy.

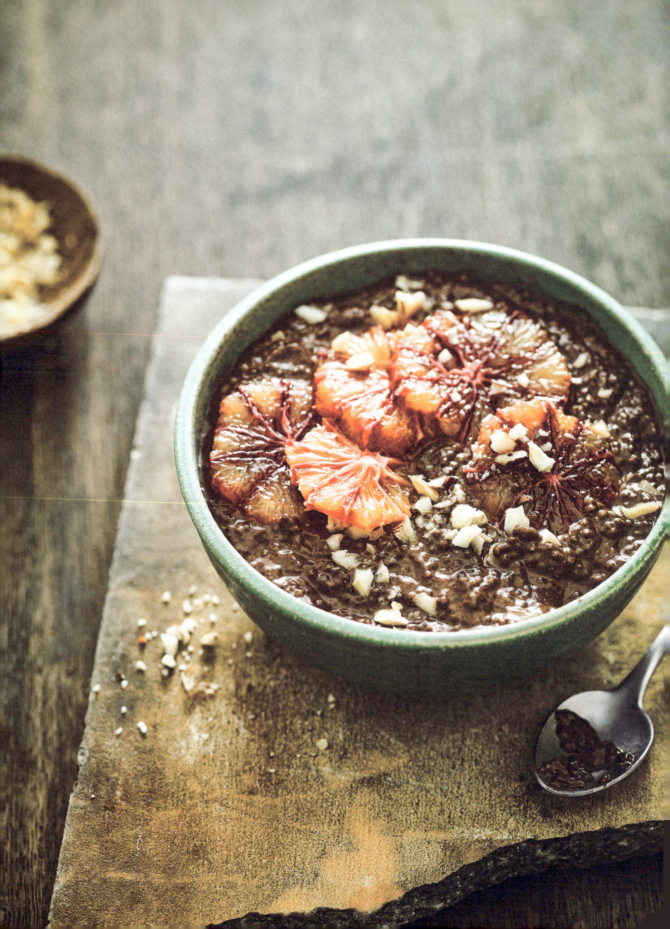

Chocolate Chia Pudding

Chia seeds have the incredible ability to create a gelatinous consistency when mixed with liquid, making them the perfect base for sweet treats that need a thick, pudding-like texture – think chocolate pudding, custard and more. And the best part? They achieve this without any added thickening agents, while packing in an impressive amount of fibre and protein. Nature really might have the answer to everything. I love snacking on this while watching a movie, satisfying my sweet tooth while treating my body right.

In a medium mixing bowl or jar, combine all the ingredients. Stir or whisk well, making sure there are no lumps of cocoa powder.

Cover the bowl or jar and place in the fridge for 3–4 hours. The chia seeds will absorb the liquid and create a thick, creamy texture.

After chilling, give the pudding a good stir to ensure a smooth consistency. If the pudding is too thick, add a little more milk (1–2 tablespoons) and stir.

Divide the pudding between serving bowls or jars. Add your favourite toppings, such as fresh fruit, coconut flakes, chopped nuts, or a drizzle of nut butter for added flavour and texture.

340ml (11½fl oz/1½ cups) unsweetened milk of choice (coconut works well)
40g (1½oz/heaped ¼ cup) chia seeds
2 tbsp cocoa powder (preferably unsweetened)
2–3 tbsp maple syrup (adjust to taste)
½ tsp ground cinnamon

Toppings (optional)
Fresh fruit
Coconut flakes
Chopped nuts
Nut butter

Notes
The sweetness can be adjusted to your taste by adding more or less maple syrup. This pudding can be made ahead and stored in the refrigerator for up to 4–5 days, making it a convenient breakfast or snack option. Feel free to experiment with different flavours by adding ground cinnamon, coffee, or even a touch of vanilla extract.

Date Caramel

Makes 250ml (9fl oz/generous 1 cup)
Prep 5 minutes

Did you know that you can blend dates and a pinch of salt with milk to create a natural date caramel? Today, living in a way that truly promotes health requires conscious, creative choices to reimagine what we've been taught about food and cooking. This date caramel is a perfect example of transformation through creation. It's the art of improvisation. With just a few whole, natural ingredients, you've got a delicious, nutrient-rich treat to satisfy your sweet cravings. A win-win.

In a high-speed blender or food processor, combine all the ingredients. Blend until smooth, ensuring no chunks of date remain. If the mixture is too thick, add more milk, 1–2 tablespoons at a time, blending after each addition, until the desired consistency is reached.

Use immediately as a topping, dip, or spread, or transfer to an airtight container and store in the fridge for up to 1 week or in the freezer for up to 3 months. Defrost before using.

16 medjool dates, pitted
1 tsp flaked sea salt
1 tsp ground cinnamon
240ml (9fl oz/1 cup) almond or
  coconut milk

Notes
For the best results, use soft medjool dates. If your dates are dry or firm, soak them in warm water for 30 minutes, then drain and proceed as above.

SWEET

Smashed Walnut & Caramel Bites

Makes 9
Prep 10 minutes, plus freezing

If there's one thing I always keep stocked, it's dates. They're nature's candy – chewy, sweet and packed with nutrients. Paired with creamy tahini, rich dark chocolate and a sprinkle of sea salt, they turn into something that tastes almost too indulgent to be this simple. But that's the beauty of real food – it doesn't take much to create something incredible. Keep these in the freezer for when the sweet cravings hit.

9 medjool dates, pitted
9 tbsp tahini (or almond butter)
100g (3½oz) dark (bittersweet) chocolate, melted
Pinch of flaked sea salt
Handful of crushed walnuts

Press each date flat using the bottom of a glass.

Spoon a generous amount of tahini (or almond butter) onto each flattened date.

Drizzle melted dark chocolate over the top, making sure each one is fully covered.

Sprinkle the dates with a pinch of sea salt and top with crushed walnuts for extra crunch.

Transfer to the freezer for about 1–2 hours until firm.

Enjoy straight from the freezer for a rich, chewy and deeply satisfying treat.

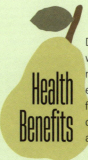

Health Benefits

Dates aren't just sweet, they're packed with natural fibre and essential minerals which leads to slow-release energy. Tahini adds a dose of healthy fats and plant-based calcium, while dark chocolate provides polyphenols and antioxidants.

Protein Chocolate Mousse

Serves 2–3
Prep 10 minutes, plus chilling

Chocolate mousse made from tofu? It's hard to believe, but it's so rich and decadent! Even though I make this all the time, I'm still shocked by how creamy and perfectly whipped it becomes after setting in the fridge. The almond butter and dark chocolate take centre stage, creating an ultra-satisfying dessert. Even better, thanks to the tofu, this is packed with an impressive amount of protein

In a high-speed blender or food processor, combine all the ingredients. Blend until smooth and creamy, scraping down the sides, as needed.

Transfer the mixture into jars or small bowls and place in the fridge for 1–2 hours to set. The longer it chills, the richer and more decadent it will become.

Top with frozen berries and grated dark chocolate, if you like, and serve chilled.

300g (10½oz) silken tofu
2 tbsp maple syrup
1 tbsp almond butter
1 tbsp cacao powder
100g (3½oz) dark (bittersweet) chocolate, melted, plus more to decorate
Frozen berries of your choice (optional), to decorate

Note

Use high-quality dark (bittersweet) chocolate with a minimum of 70 per cent cocoa solids. This ensures a rich taste and provides more antioxidants while minimising added sugar.

SWEET

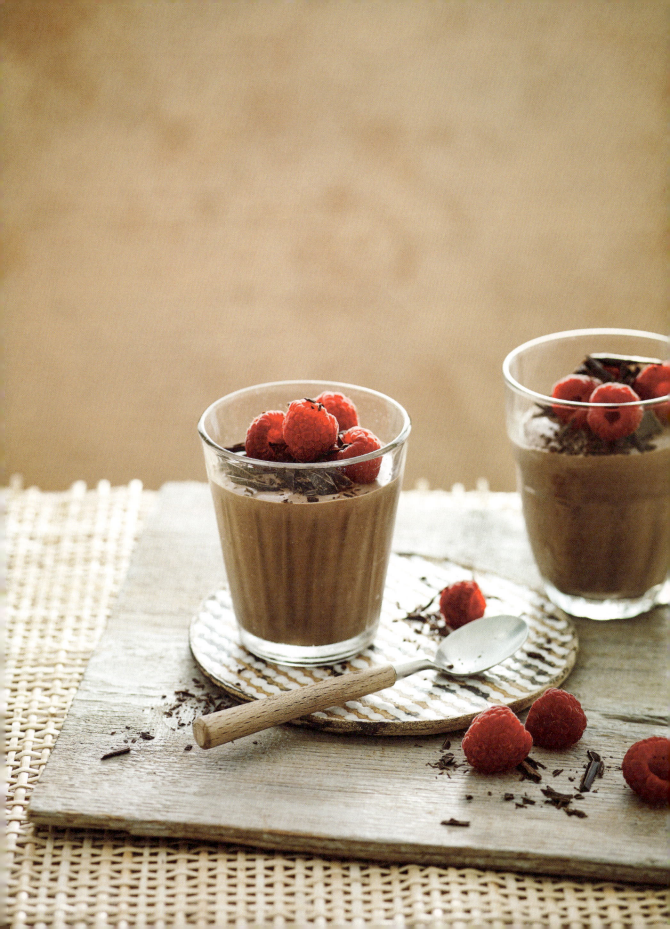

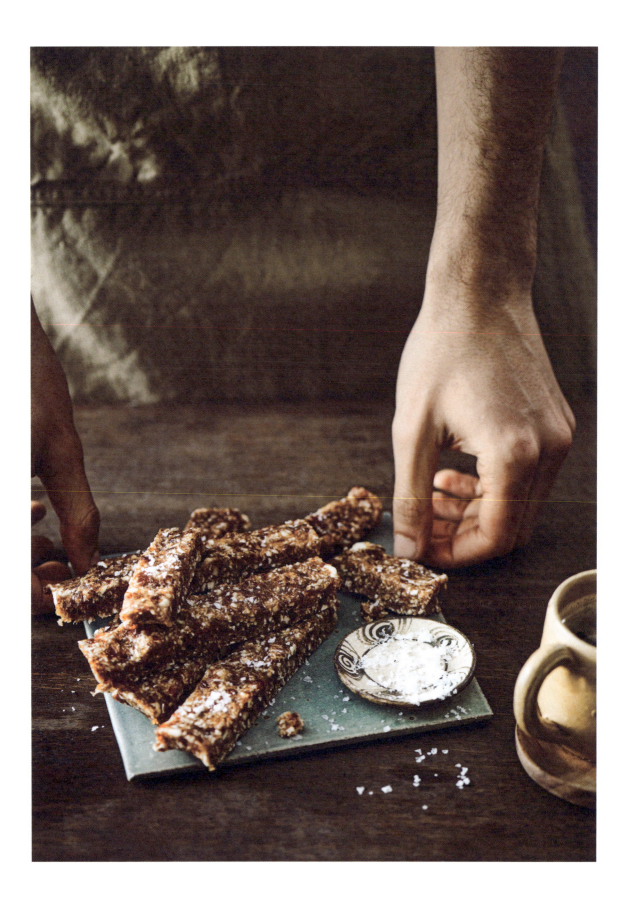

Crunchy Almond Bliss Snacks

Makes 8–10

Prep 3 minutes

I remember walking through the grocery aisles with my younger siblings, their eyes glued to the flashy snack packaging. I tried to explain that the front of the packaging is for entertainment, but the back is where the truth lies. Although, reading out the endless ingredients in a 'kid-friendly' coconut cereal didn't seem to bother them much. One thing kids love, however, is a challenge. So, I challenged us to make our own cereal-like snacks with just a handful of unprocessed ingredients. To this day, it's still their favourite quick sweet treat.

350g (12oz) medjool dates, pitted
75g (2¾oz) almonds
40g (1½oz/½ cup) desiccated (dried shredded) coconut
Pinch of sea salt

In a high-speed blender or food processor, combine the dates, almonds, desiccated coconut and sea salt. Blend on low until the mixture resembles coarse crumbs and begins to stick together.

Transfer it to a small dish or tin lined with parchment paper. Press down firmly using your hands or the back of a spoon until evenly compacted.

Place in the fridge for at least 1 hour to firm up, then slice into small bars or squares.

Store in an airtight container in the fridge for up to 2 weeks.

Tropical Nice Cream

Craving something sweet? Your body is actually asking for energy, and this ice cream is the ultimate way to satisfy that craving while fuelling yourself with real nourishment. Unlike processed sugars that spike and crash your energy, the natural sugars in bananas and mangoes are packed with nutrients that support vitality, digestion and even mood. Bananas are nature's perfect sweetener, loaded with antioxidants, B vitamins and gut-loving prebiotics that keep digestion running smoothly. Mangoes bring a dose of vitamin C and immune-boosting compounds. Together, they create a creamy, dreamy dessert that feels like indulgence but is actually working *for* you. Whether you enjoy this as a refreshing snack, a dessert, or even a nourishing breakfast, this is one scoop you'll always feel good about.

In a food processor or high-speed blender, combine the banana, mango and vanilla extract. Pulse a few times to break everything down, then blend continuously. If needed, add a splash of coconut water or plant milk, 1 tablespoon at a time, until a thick, creamy texture is reached.

Serve immediately for a soft-serve texture, or freeze for 30 minutes to firm up. Scoop into bowls and enjoy as is, or top with coconut flakes, fresh berries, or a drizzle of tahini for extra depth.

4 frozen bananas, cut into chunks
225g (8oz) frozen mango chunks
1 tsp vanilla extract
A splash of coconut water or plant milk, if needed

Toppings (optional)
Coconut flakes
Fresh berries
Tahini

Notes
The key to getting that perfect creamy texture? Frozen fruit. Using frozen bananas and mangos is what gives this its thick, scoopable consistency. Fresh fruit just won't blend the same way, so make sure your bananas are fully frozen before blending.

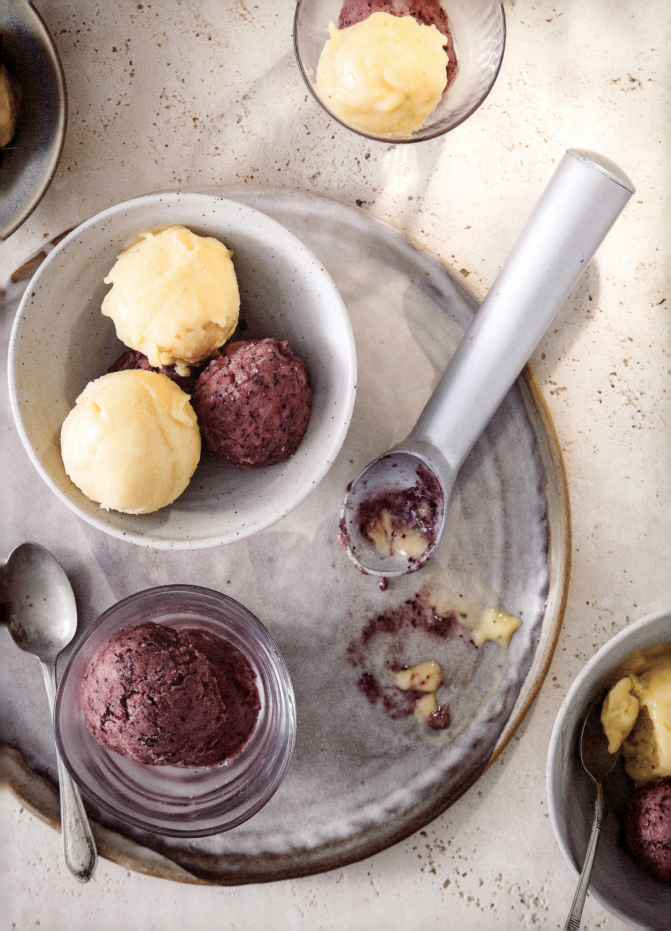

Brain Fuel: Blueberry Nice Cream

Serves 3–4
Prep 5 minutes

Your brain deserves the best fuel. Blueberries aren't just a delicious fruit – they're one of the most powerful foods for brain health. They boost cognitive function and even aid in emotional balance. Wild blueberries are smaller but pack in more flavour and nutrients than regular blueberries. They contain up to twice the antioxidants, more fibre and grow naturally without pesticides. If you have access to them, they're the better choice for both taste and nutrition. This isn't just ice cream – it's a spoonful of deep nourishment for the mind and body. Blended with frozen bananas for natural creaminess, this Blueberry Nice Cream is a refreshing, nutrient-dense treat that satisfies cravings while delivering serious health benefits. With just a few ingredients and no dairy or processed sugars, it is pure, healing goodness.

In a high-speed blender or food processor, combine the frozen banana pieces and frozen blueberries. Pulse a few times to break them down, then blend continuously, scraping down the sides as needed.

Add 1–2 tablespoons of water or milk, if needed, to help it blend smoothly, but avoid adding too much – you want it thick and creamy.

Add the raw honey or date syrup for extra sweetness, if using, then blend again until fully combined.

Serve immediately for a soft-serve texture, or transfer to a freezer-safe container and freeze for 30 minutes for a firmer consistency.

5 frozen bananas, chopped into pieces

225g (8oz) frozen blueberries (ideally wild blueberries)

1–2 tbsp unsweetened milk of choice (coconut or almond work well) or water, if needed

1 tsp raw honey or date syrup (optional)

Note

Wild blueberries are one of the most healing foods on the planet – their powerful antioxidants remove toxins and promote the growth of new, healthy brain cells. If you're feeling foggy, stressed, or mentally drained, this is the kind of nourishment your brain craves.

The Gladiator's Muffin

Makes 12
Prep 10 minutes
Cook 30 minutes

The Ancient Egyptians and Roman gladiators knew what they were doing when they relied on spelt – a grain packed with fibre, protein and nutrients that fuelled them through battle and hard labour. Today, we're still catching on to how powerful these ancient grains really are. These muffins bring together spelt's nutty depth with the natural sweetness of ripe pears and bananas, balanced by warm cinnamon, nutmeg and ginger, which support digestion and blood sugar balance. They're soft, subtly spiced and naturally sweet – proof that a treat doesn't have to slow you down. No highly processed ingredients, no nonsense – just real food that tastes as good as it makes you feel.

Preheat the oven to Fan 160°C/180°C/350°F/Gas 6 and line a 12-hole muffin tin with paper cases.

In a large mixing bowl, combine the flour, date or coconut sugar, bicarbonate of soda, baking powder, cinnamon, nutmeg, ginger and a pinch of sea salt, and mix until well combined.

In a separate bowl, combine the mashed bananas, milk, melted coconut oil and tahini (or almond butter), mixing until fully incorporated.

Pour the wet ingredients into the dry ingredients and mix gently until combined. Fold in the chopped pears, making sure they're evenly distributed.

Spoon 2–3 tablespoons of batter into each muffin case. You could add sliced pears, crushed walnuts, or pistachios to top of each muffin, if liked, then sprinkle with some more cinnamon and nutmeg.

Bake in the preheated oven for 20–30 minutes, or until the muffins turn golden and a knife inserted into the centre comes out clean.

Set aside to cool for 5–10 minutes, then enjoy. Soft, spiced and naturally sweet – these will be your new go-to treat.

230g (8oz/1¾ cups) white spelt flour
200g (7oz) date sugar (or coconut sugar)
1 tsp bicarbonate of soda (baking soda)
½ tsp baking powder
1 tsp ground cinnamon, plus extra to top
½ tsp ground nutmeg, plus extra to top
½ tsp ground ginger
Pinch of sea salt
3 ripe bananas, mashed
4 tbsp unsweetened milk of choice (coconut or almond work well)
3 tbsp coconut oil, melted
2 tbsp tahini (or almond butter)
2 pears, peeled and diced

Toppings (optional)
Sliced banana
Crushed walnuts or pistachios

Note
Spelt flour works best for this recipe – it keeps the muffins light, moist and full of flavour. While buckwheat or other gluten-free flours can be used, they don't hold the same structure or depth of flavour, making the muffins denser and less balanced.

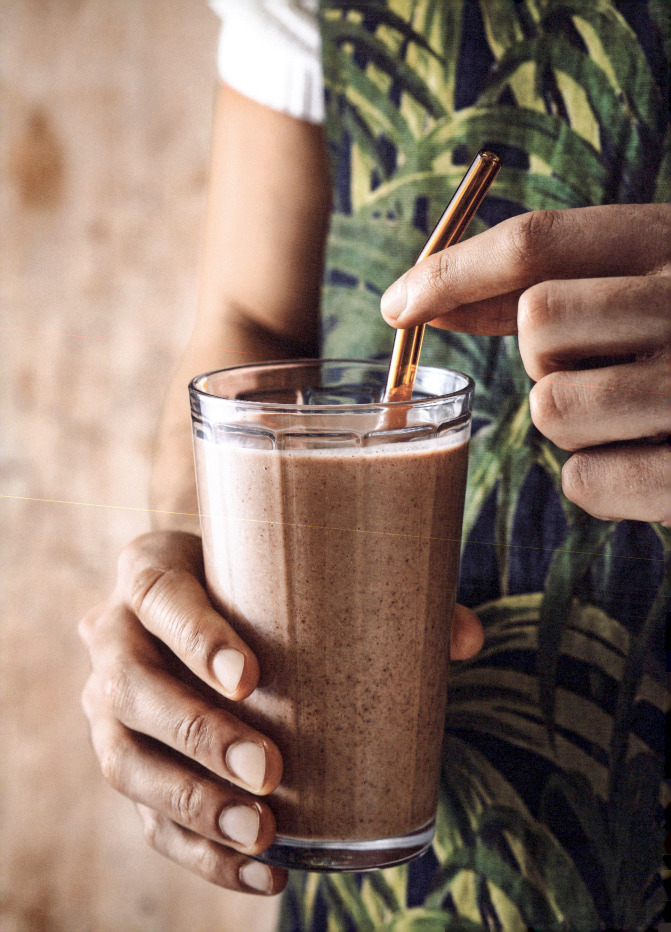

Crunch the Cravings

Serves 1–2

Prep 2 minutes

Sweetness is more than just a craving – it's the body's way of seeking comfort, warmth and connection. Sometimes, what we really need isn't just food, but nourishment that soothes the soul. Processed sugar gives a quick high but leaves you drained. Nature's candy – bananas, dates and cinnamon – gives that same sweetness but in a form your body recognises and thrives on. This smoothie is thick, creamy and naturally indulgent, blended with warming spices and almond butter for richness. It's the kind of thing that wraps around you like a warm hug, grounding you while satisfying every craving.

5 medjool dates, pitted

2 ripe bananas, halved

3 tbsp almond butter

325ml (11fl oz/1⅓ cups) unsweetened milk of choice (coconut or almond work well)

1 tsp ground cinnamon

Pinch of ground cloves

1 tsp raw cacao powder (optional)

In a high-speed blender or food processor, combine all the ingredients. Blend until smooth. Let it run for 30–60 seconds, scraping down the sides, if needed, until you get a thick, creamy consistency. Adjust as needed: if you like it thicker, add a few ice cubes or some frozen banana; if you prefer it thinner, add a splash more milk.

Pour and enjoy immediately for the freshest taste – creamy, spiced and naturally sweet.

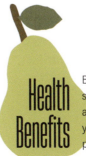

Health Benefits

Bananas and dates bring natural sweetness alongside fibre, potassium and slow-releasing energy to keep you steady. Almond butter adds protein and healthy fats.

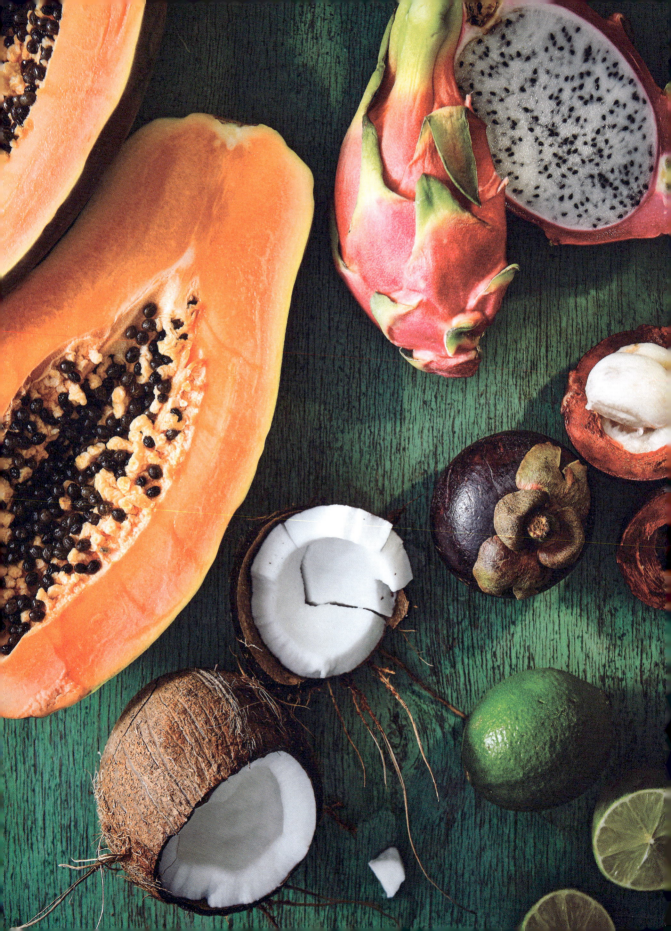

THE 30-DAY CHALLENGE

Weekly Meal Planners

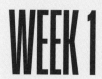

	Breakfast	Lunch	Dinner	Snack
Monday	Deep Comfort Cacao Porridge p.40	Chickpea Omelette p.69	The Earth Bowl p.93	Raw Power Bites p.173
Tuesday	Deep Comfort Cacao Porridge p.40	Chickpea Omelette p.69	The Earth Bowl p.93	Raw Power Bites p.173
Wednesday	Breakfast Vitality Blend p.50	To-Go 20-Minute Power Bowl p.75	Tofu Bolognese p.104	Raw Power Bites p.173
Thursday	Breakfast Vitality Blend p.50	To-Go 20-Minute Power Bowl p.75	Tofu Bolognese p.104	Smashed Snickers Bites p.177
Friday	Green Goodness Smoothie p.30	15-Minute Power Beans p.72	The Go-To Dal p.96	Smashed Snickers Bites p.177
Saturday	Green Goodness Smoothie p.30	15-Minute Power Beans p.72	The Go-To Dal p.96	Smashed Snickers Bites p.177
Sunday	Gut-Friendly Pancakes p.45	Chickpea Protein Smoothie p.67	Power Black Bean Stew p.102	Apple Pie in a Glass p.166

WEEK 2

	Breakfast	Lunch	Dinner	Snack
Monday	Gut-Friendly Pancakes p.45	Chickpea Protein Smoothie p.67	Power Black Bean Stew p.102	Apple Pie in a Glass p.166
Tuesday	Tofu Scramble p.46	My Sister's Everyday Glow Salad p.71	Chilli p.112	Crunchy Almond Bliss Snacks p.181
Wednesday	Tofu Scramble p.46	My Sister's Everyday Glow Salad p.71	Chilli p.112	Crunchy Almond Bliss Snacks p.181
Thursday	Creamy Weight Gain Smoothie p.59	Edamame Power Smash p.78	Broccoli & Butter Bean Power Stir p.90	Crunchy Almond Bliss Snacks p.181
Friday	Creamy Weight Gain Smoothie p.59	Edamame Power Smash p.78	Broccoli & Butter Bean Power Stir p.90	Tropical Nice Cream p.182
Saturday	Quinoa Porridge p.38	Chuna p.76	Rustic Tuscan Bean & Kale Soup p.116	Tropical Nice Cream p.182
Sunday	Quinoa Porridge p.38	Chuna p.76	Rustic Tuscan Bean & Kale Soup p.116	Tropical Nice Cream p.182

WEEK 3

	Breakfast	Lunch	Dinner	Snack
Monday	Green Smoothie Bowl p.34	To-Go 20-Minute Power Bowl p.75	Chickpea Curry p.115	Whole fruits
Tuesday	Green Smoothie Bowl p.34	To-Go 20-Minute Power Bowl p.75	Chickpea Curry p.115	Whole fruits
Wednesday	Chocolate Chickpea Pancakes p.43	Roasted Tomato & Cashew Soup p.84	Loaded Sweet Potato p.99	Whole fruits
Thursday	Chocolate Chickpea Pancakes p.43	Roasted Tomato & Cashew Soup p.84	Loaded Sweet Potato p.99	Crunch the Cravings p.187
Friday	Nutty Heaven p.54	Glow-Up Pesto p.84	The Nourishment Bowl p.94	Crunch the Cravings p.187
Saturday	Nutty Heaven p.54	Glow-Up Pesto p.84	The Nourishment Bowl p.94	Crunch the Cravings p.187
Sunday	Mango Lassi p.55	Chickpea Omelette p.69	Meaty Mushroom Stew p.104	Protein Chocolate Mousse p.178

WEEK 4

	Breakfast	Lunch	Dinner	Snack
Monday	Mango Lassi p.55	Chickpea Omelette p.69	Meaty Mushroom Stew p.101	Protein Chocolate Mousse p.178
Tuesday	Creamy Power Porridge p.37	Nourishing Broccoli Soup p.62	The Lentil Stew You Won't Forget p.118	Protein Chocolate Mousse p.178
Wednesday	Creamy Power Porridge p.37	Nourishing Broccoli Soup p.62	The Lentil Stew You Won't Forget p.118	Cinnamon Baked Pear p.170
Thursday	Salted Caramel Smoothie Bowl p.33	15-Minute Power Beans p.72	Comforting Chickpea Noodle Soups p.114	Cinnamon Baked Pear p.170
Friday	Salted Caramel Smoothie Bowl p.33	15-Minute Power Beans p.72	Comforting Chickpea Noodle Soups p.114	Cinnamon Baked Pear p.170
Saturday	Chickpea Scramble p.51	Edamame Power Smash p.78	Smoky Chipotle-Spiced Tofu p.88	Gluten-Free Sweet Potato Brownies p.162
Sunday	Chickpea Scramble p.51	Edamame Power Smash p.78	Smoky Chipotle-Spiced Tofu p.88	Gluten-Free Sweet Potato Brownies p.162

Clean Eating Lifestyle Tips

[1]   Set Your Environment Up for Success

Just like a lion in the wild conserves energy by resting for most of the day, we instinctively seek the path of least resistance, too. If there's junk food within arm's reach, it's only natural to reach for it. If ultra-processed snacks are stocked in your kitchen, they will be the easiest option. The key to long-term success isn't willpower – it's creating an environment that supports your goals.

Make clean eating the most accessible choice. Swap out processed snacks for fresh fruits, raw nuts and naturally sweet options, like dates stuffed with almond butter and a sprinkle of sea salt. Replace sugary energy drinks with coconut water or lemon-infused water. When healthy choices are the default, convenience no longer comes at the cost of long-term health.

[2]   Cook In Batches

Nature thrives on preparation – just like a squirrel gathers food ahead of winter, we can apply the same strategy to our daily lives. When hunger strikes, convenience wins, and the easiest choice often becomes the default. The key to making eating whole food effortless is having nourishing meals ready to go. Cooking in batches saves time, energy and effort throughout the week. Double up on soups, stews and grains, so that a nutrient-dense meal is always within reach. Roast a tray of vegetables, boil sweet potatoes in bulk, and keep staple ingredients prepped in the fridge. Most evenings, all I do is reheat a stew, warm up my carbs, slice an avocado and throw in some leafy greens. This significantly reduces daily preparation time and works in alignment with our innate mechanisms of conserving energy. With a little foresight, clean eating becomes second nature.

[3]   The Blueprint – Structuring Your Week

Planning ahead is one of the simplest ways to stay on track. A structured weekly rhythm of eating not only takes the guesswork out of mealtime but also ensures your kitchen is stocked with the right ingredients, making clean eating effortless. Instead of scrambling for last-minute options, you'll have nourishing meals ready to go, reducing the temptation to fall back on processed foods. Start the day with a clear plan – know exactly what your breakfast consists of, what ingredients it requires and how long it takes to prepare. This greatly reduces the likelihood of grabbing ultra-processed alternatives on the go. For some, repetition is key. Sticking to the same meal throughout the week can simplify things when time is limited. Your go-to could be the Quinoa Porridge or the Green Goodness Smoothie – meals that provide steady energy and set the tone for the day ahead.

Think of this as more than a weekly menu, it's a system designed to fuel you, freeing up time and mental energy so that nourishing yourself becomes effortless.

[4]   Stay Ready, Stay Nourished

Life moves fast and when hunger hits, having something ready to grab can make all the difference. Just like a bird instinctively gathers food before a long journey, we can set ourselves up for success by preparing in advance. A simple 'to-go box' filled with nutrient-dense snacks can prevent you from relying on processed options when you're out and about.

Keep a small container or reusable bag stocked with whole food essentials – nuts, seeds, dried fruit, homemade energy balls, or a small jar of nut butter with apple slices. Some of my favourites include cashews, dates and Brazil nuts, cooked chestnuts, or apple slices with tahini. Having real food within reach means you're less likely to make impulsive choices that don't serve your long-term well-being. Preparation is key, and something as small as a pre-packed snack can keep you on track, no matter where the day takes you.

[5]   Community & Support

Food is meant to be shared. Throughout history, meals have brought people together, strengthening bonds and building community. Preparing whole food meals doesn't have to be a solo mission – getting help makes the process easier, more enjoyable and more sustainable. One of the greatest joys of embracing this lifestyle was sharing newly discovered recipes with my sister – and her doing the same with me. It wasn't just about the food, it deepened our bond and, over time, became the source of a collection of recipes suited to every occasion.

If you share a household, involve those around you – assign tasks, batch-cook together, or simply ask for support so you have your family or housemates on board with your journey. If you live alone, consider meal prepping with a friend or becoming part of an online community.

And beyond the kitchen, don't hesitate to seek guidance – whether that's learning from books, online resources, or health-conscious communities. We thrive when we lean on each other, and making clean eating a shared effort ensures the experience is all the more rewarding and joyful.

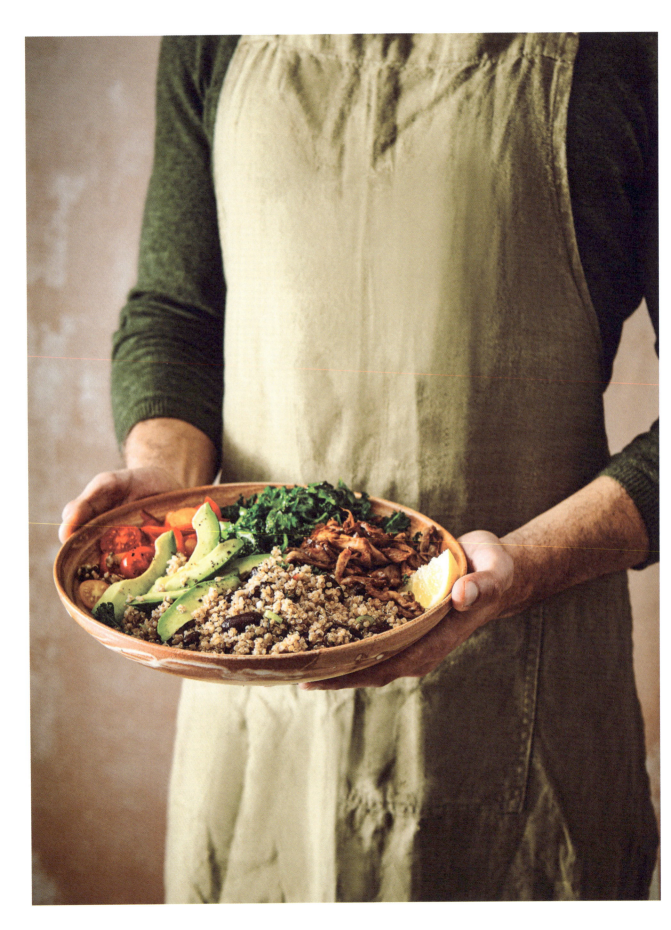

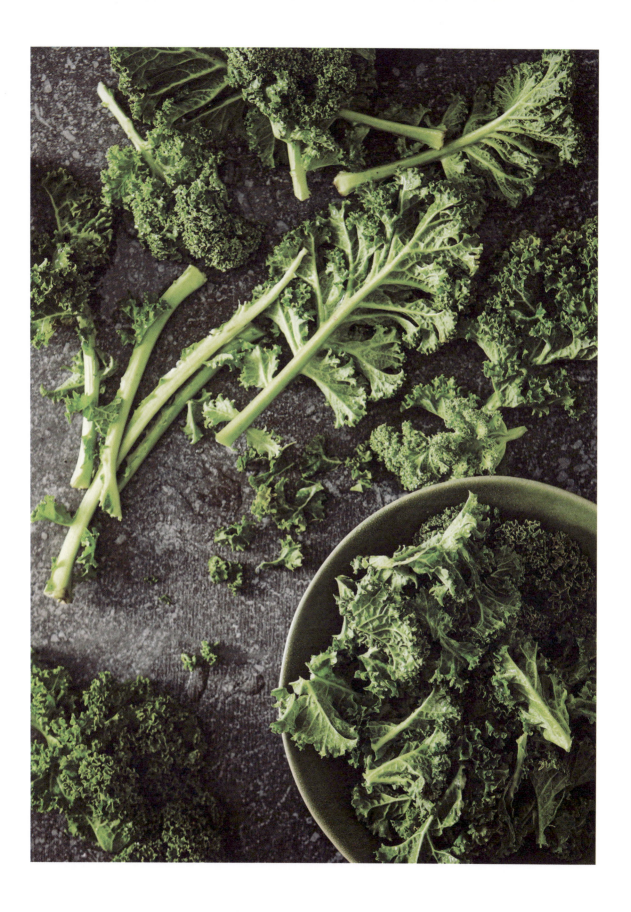

AFTER THE 30 DAYS: WHAT NEXT?

By now, something has shifted. Not just in your body – though you may be feeling lighter, more energised and deeply nourished – but in your relationship with food. You've seen how real food can recalibrate the way you feel, the way you move, the way you think. You've proven something to yourself: that it is possible to live well without the labels, the processed noise, or the pull of convenience culture. And it starts on your plate.

So, what now?

This isn't where the journey ends. It's where it begins again – not as a challenge, but as a lifestyle. One that is sustainable, rooted and aligned. A way of eating, living and choosing that aligns with how you want to feel in your body and in your life. These past 30 days were never about a finish line. They were about remembering: how to listen to your body, how to feed it what it truly needs and how to trust its response.

From here, it's about carrying that knowing forward in a way that fits into your life. You might not eat this way every single day, and that's okay, life is fluid, but the awareness that you've cultivated is something you carry forward. A new internal compass. Now, you know what makes you feel good. You know the difference between feeling full and feeling nourished. You'll sense when your body is calling for greens, hydration, simplicity and you'll trust that knowledge, because you've experienced the difference.

Some days, you might lean into a hearty bowl of lentils and roasted roots. Other days, it might be a fresh juice, a handful of nuts, or a wild swim that resets you. This isn't about rules, it's about rhythm.

Here are some ways to keep the momentum going:

- **Revisit your favourites.** Which meals made you feel most alive? Which routines supported you best? Prioritise those and build on them. There's no need to reinvent your plate every week – consistency is a form of care.

- **Stay curious.** Explore new ingredients. Visit local farmers' markets. Try a wild food walk. Nourishment doesn't have to be repetitive, it can be an adventure.

- **Check in with yourself.** This is a practice, a path. Some weeks might feel aligned and vibrant, others might feel out of step. That's natural. Just come back to what you know: how good it feels to eat in a way that honours your body.

- **Don't fall for the quick fixes again.** After 30 days of real food, it's easy to feel tempted to go back, just for a taste or for convenience, and that's okay. There's no shame in veering off path. But notice how your body responds. Use it as feedback, not failure.

- **Be flexible, not perfect.** This isn't all or nothing, it's all about balance. If you veer off-path, don't spiral, just return. The body remembers what feels good.

- **Make space for joy.** Food is not just fuel. It's connection, culture and comfort. Celebrate it and share it. Make a big pot of soup for friends, light a candle at dinner, at outside. Let nourishment be a ritual, not a restriction.

- **Honour your body's signals.** Fullness, tiredness, thirst and hunger – they're all messages. Keep tuning in. That internal compass? It's still guiding you.

You've stepped away from the processed noise and remembered what real food feels like. You've reminded your body of its natural rhythm, and now, even when you drift, that rhythm is easier to return to. You're no longer eating out of habit. You're eating with intention. And most importantly, you're in control. Not of every outcome or every craving, but of your awareness, your choices and your ability to course-correct.

So let this be your next chapter, not one driven by fear, but by freedom. Let food continue to support you, not weigh you down. Let every meal be a chance to listen and to respond. You've already done the hard part: you've said yes to change. Now keep going, keep tuning in and let this way of eating become something bigger than a challenge, let it become the beginning of something lasting.

INDEX

Further Notes

Fruits & Vegetables

The best place to source fresh, high-quality produce is your local farmer's market or farm shop. These markets offer food as close to the source as possible – seasonal, fresh and packed with the nutrients your body needs at the right time of year. They often provide organic options, ensuring minimal interference with the natural growing process.

Take the time to speak with the farmers or vendors. Understanding where your food comes from and how it was grown deepens your connection to what you eat. Most are happy to share insights about their farming practices and offer guidance on the best seasonal selections.

If you're based in London, you can find your nearest farmer's market here: https://www.lfm.org.uk/

Ancient grains, nuts, seeds & legumes

If you have access to a local organic shop, that will be one of the best places to find high-quality, nutrient-dense ingredients. These stores typically offer a wide variety of organic options.

Some of my favourite London-based shops include: Planet Organic / Whole Foods / Borough Market / Waitrose / Harvest / Daylesford Organic.

If you prefer buying in bulk or need hard-to-find ingredients, Buy Whole Foods Online is a great option for convenient online shopping.

Herbs & Supplements

Try: Buy Whole Foods Online / Amazon / Healf / The Electric Tribe.

Mushrooms

I recommend: Merit Mushrooms / Riverford Organic Farmers.

Acknowledgements

I dedicate this book to my late mother, Saskia Susanne Mackson, whose boundless love for God, her children and nature shaped the environment in which I grew up. It was one that encouraged critical thinking, the exploration of ideas and emphasised the importance of following my internal voice. Her eternal love remains present within me, guiding my every step.

My twin sister, Janine Mackson, my innate best friend, gifted to me from birth. From a young age, I have always looked up to her. Her fearless attitude toward life has inspired me to take risks, move with intention and find joy in the unknown. She has been my greatest supporter in everything I do and truly brings balance to my life. My greatest gift in this lifetime.

Finally, to my father, Michael Ola Mackson, to whom I am eternally grateful for instilling in me the core values of life. He is the embodiment of 'walk the talk' – teaching me how to nourish myself with what little we had growing up and how to care for myself physically. Through his unshakeable love and guidance, he has always provided me with protection, wisdom and support, simply by being a present and caring father.

About the Author

Jason Adetola Mackson founded The Electric Tribe in 2021 as a community created to share the recipes that helped his mother regain her health, inspire others facing cancer and to support people striving for optimal wellbeing. Through this community of over 1 million people and his health website (where they have sold over 25,000 units of vegan seaweed supplements worldwide, and become a leader in the UK) he has witnessed first-hand the power of our lifestyle choices – especially when it comes to food.

Quarto

First published in 2025 by Carnival
an imprint of The Quarto Group.
One Triptych Place, London, SE1 9SH,
United Kingdom
T (0)20 7700 9000
www.Quarto.com

EEA Representation, WTS Tax d.o.o., Žanova ulica 3, 4000 Kranj, Slovenia
www.wts-tax.si

A catalogue record for this book is available from the British Library.

ISBN 978-1-83600-961-0
Ebook ISBN 978-1-83600-962-7

10 9 8 7 6 5 4 3 2 1

Design by Georgie Hewitt

Publisher: Eleanor Maxfield
Senior Designer: Isabel Eeles
Senior Editors: Nicky Hill and Charlotte Frost
Senior Production Controller: Rohana Yusof

Printed in Guangdong, China TT092025

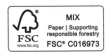

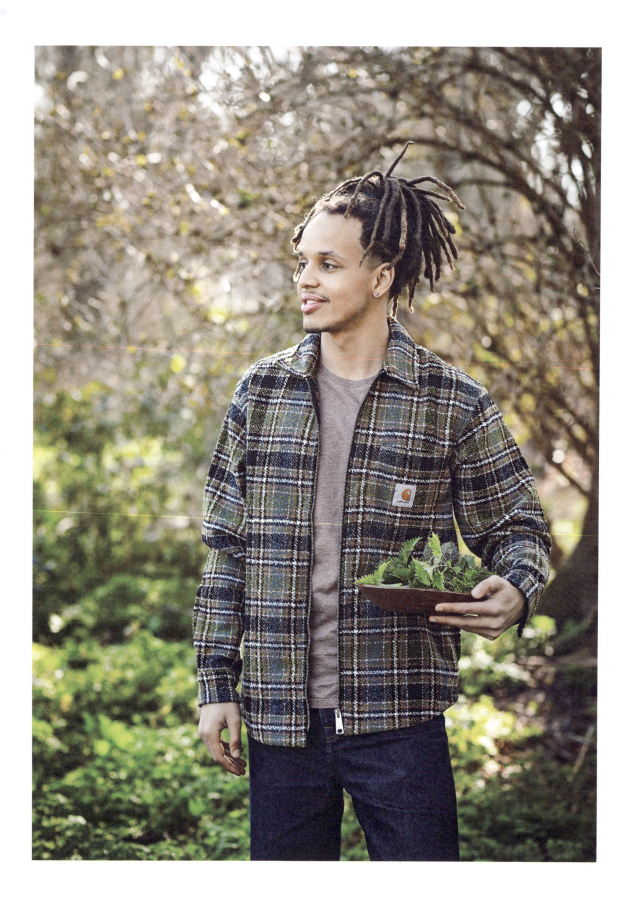